For Ashley and Emily where it all began…

With so much gratitude to Nusse, Suzie, Doris, Allison, Uta,
Matthew, Kris and Troels, for supporting me to write this.
And to Gordon and Wylde for teaching me.
And, ultimately and kinda most importantly my thanks to Julie
for saving my life so I actually got to write this.

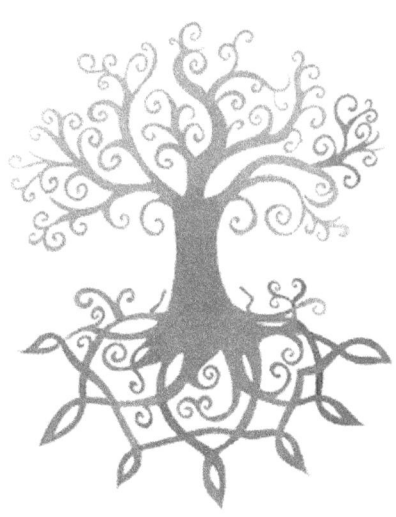

'When you need it, nature is there to guide you. Whether in the roots of the trees, the crevices in the stone, the foam on the wave or the scent in the wind. You are a part of nature. Nature is your wisest teacher and you're ... nature's guardian. As she supports us, we take care of her. So we can grow together, dancing to the rhythm of life, the heartbeat of the earth ...'

– From *Walking the Wheel of the Year*.

Table of Contents

Introduction	7
The Wheel of the Year	9
Getting Started	12
Samhain	15
Yule and the Winter Solstice	31
Imbolc	49
Ostara and the Spring Equinox	67
Beltane	93
Litha and the Summer Solstice	113
Lammas	137
Mabon and the Autumn Equinox	161
Samhain the Ending and the Beginning	185
Walking the Wheel of the Year from Now on	201
Additional Resources	202
The Tree of Life – the gateway to connection	203
Recommended reading	207
Bibliography	209

Introduction

Welcome to your *Walking the Wheel of the Year* companion workbook! At the end of the *Walking the Wheel of the Year* book, I passed your journey back to you: 'From here on in, you lead your journey.' And you absolutely do. However, I know from my own early days of aligning my life to the Wheel of the Year; despite being incredibly inspiring, it was also a little overwhelming. It can seem a lot, right? Eight festivals a year: internal work, connection work, ceremonies, journeys, crafting and celebrations. And everyday life as well! I remember all too well how daunting it felt to me. And that daunting, overwhelming feeling can be a block to us even starting our journey of aligning and connecting with nature's rhythms.

And to that I say, 'Hell. No!' (Pardon my language.)

My dream has always been to make re-rooting in yourself, re-rooting with nature's seasons and aligning with the Wheel of the Year as accessible as possible, to as many people as possible. Which is why I have been inspired to create this companion workbook – to support you on your first steps, or possibly your deeper steps, on the magical lifestyle that is to live aligned with nature and create your own spiritual path.

Walking the Wheel of the Year is not just about celebrating the festivals; it is about aligning your life with the journey of the wheel. I often say in my workshops that the festivals of the wheel give us a moment to pause and do the deeper reflections; however, it is in between the festivals that we do the work. And in this workbook you have space to do both. To take the moments to pause, to re-root, to connect, to celebrate and to continue your growth throughout the wheel. By choosing this book, you are already saying to yourself, to the universe, I am ready, I want to find my path; to nature, I want to be part of your cycle; and to yourself, I am ready to nourish my roots, accept, love, empower myself and grow. And how you will! I am excited for you and I hope you are too.

Now, before we begin, there are some important things to cover about using this workbook. Firstly, and most importantly, as I said in *Walking the Wheel of the Year*, you do what feels right for you. Take what works for you and leave the rest behind. One Samhain, you may want to really look into your ancestors; at another, you may find that you are more focused on letting go. And that is completely ok. We need different things to nourish us in the different stages of our lives. Let your instinct guide you, and don't fill your heads with 'shoulds'. There is no specific way you 'should' be connecting with nature. There are no 'shoulds' in nature. If there were, evolution wouldn't happen. So I am going to be a little bit strict and say you are not allowed to feel bad that you didn't do every exercise in this workbook, this wheel or the next. Do what feels right and what you can.

Secondly, you don't have to wait until Samhain to start using this workbook. As much as it is lovely to start your journey with the wheel at Samhain, you don't have to. The first festival I ever celebrated was Imbolc. So, if you have picked this book up at Beltane or Mabon, you can start now. The only thing I would say is that the first year, you start with the first Samhain exercise, not the last. There is a lot going on at Samhain – so much so that in the book I have split it into two. After your first year using this workbook, you can use whichever parts of Samhain you like. Again, follow your gut and do what is right for you.

And did I say the 'first time' you use this book? Yes, I did. The last important thing I suggest is to fill this book in using a pencil. That way you will be able to not only reflect on the previous year's journey, but you can also use this book continuously.

I won't take any more of your time with my musings. Except to say thank you for allowing me the gift of supporting you on this journey.

My love and blessings to you,

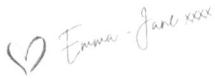

The Wheel of the Year

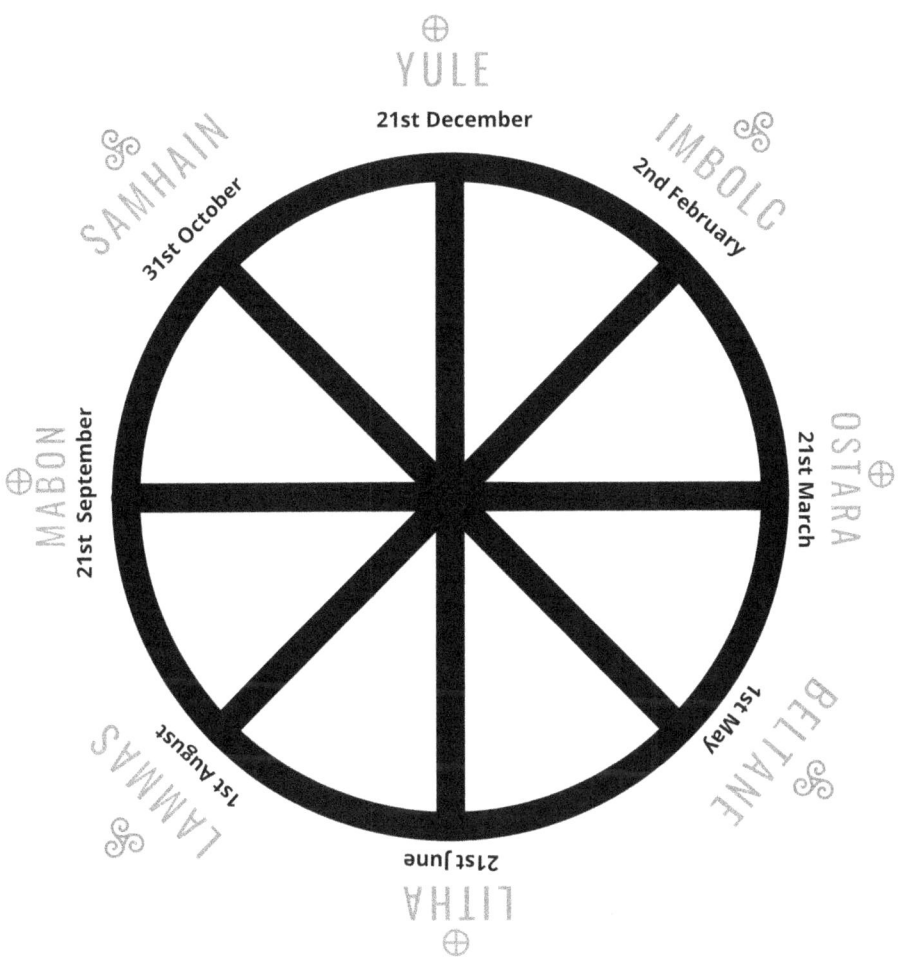

WHAT IS THE WHEEL OF THE YEAR?

SAMHAIN (October 31) (Fire Festival)
Samhain represents the final harvest before the long winter. It is a celebration of death, an acceptance that all life must die so that life can be created once more. It is a time to honor our ancestors and embrace the darker half of the year. This also marks the beginning of the Celtic New Year, when the seasons die to be reborn again.

Walking the Wheel of the Year themes:
Where we came from, our ancestors, letting go, and the last harvest.

YULE/MIDWINTER SOLSTICE (December 20–23)
Yule marks the winter solstice, the longest night and the shortest day of the year. A time of celebration of surviving the cold dark times, and storytelling through the darkest night. From here, at dawn we celebrate the sun's rebirth…

Walking the Wheel of the Year themes:
Where we are now, the gifts of those we love, the sacred child, and the birth of the summer sun.

IMBOLC (February 2) (Fire Festival)
Imbolc is a festival of fire and light. It marks the time when the first shoots are starting to appear, the buds are just beginning to open. This is a festival of purification, a festival of light, inspiration and new beginnings. Imbolc is also called Candlemas, and it was the time when new candles were made.

Walking the Wheel of the Year themes:
Inspiration, new beginnings, hopes and dreams.

OSTARA/SPRING EQUINOX (March 20–23)
Ostara is the celebration of the spring equinox. A point of balance. Day and night are equal. The animals are birthing their young

and awakening from their winter sleep. Here we move from the dark half of the year and into the light.

Walking the Wheel of the Year themes:
Balance, manifestation, and the shadow self.

BELTANE (May 1) (Fire Festival)
Beltane celebrates the fertility of the earth and man. It is a time of love, passion, fire, dance and abundance. Beltane is when we connect to the heartbeat of the earth.

Walking the Wheel of the Year themes:
How we can better love and honour ourselves, stepping into a place of self love.

LITHA/MIDSUMMER SOLSTICE (June 20–23)
Litha, the summer solstice, is the longest day of the year and the shortest night. It's a celebration of the height of the sun's power – from here onwards, the days become shorter.

Walking the Wheel of the Year themes:
How we can step into our most powerful self and learn how to connect with that self when we need to.

LAMMAS (August 1) (Fire Festival)
Lammas is the first harvest festival. This is a time of celebrating the abundance of the first harvest and community.

Walking the Wheel of the Year themes:
The first harvest, gratitude and community.

MABON/AUTUMN EQUINOX (September 20–23)
Mabon is a time of thanksgiving celebrating the berry harvest and the autumnal equinox. It is a time of balance. Day and night are equal. It is a time of preparation where we gather exactly the sweet things we need to sustain us through winter.

Walking the Wheel of the Year themes:
The sweet harvest, abundance, pride and honouring our light.

Getting Started

CREATE A SACRED SPACE

Your journey with the wheel is not just outside, it is inside too. Inside you, of course, but also inside your home.

Dedicating an area of your home to your spiritual journey is a powerful way of keeping your journey at the forefront of your mind. It does not need to be fancy, but it does need to be somewhere you can decorate – a surface, a shelf, or even a windowsill. Throughout my journey, I've always had such a space. From my first little altar on top of a bookshelf, made with cardboard boxes and gaffa tape and decorated with a pretty scarf, and the thin shelf above my gas fireplace, to the beautiful wooden dresser that takes central space in my office today – there's always a part of my home dedicated to mine and nature's journey. By creating a space that you can decorate with nature for the season, you will be physically connecting with the wheel and inviting nature into your home.

You can decorate your space any way you like. There are no hard and fast rules. And keep it simple. Simple is very important and, most of all, personal. The objects decorating your space need to be important to you.

One thing that I love to do as the wheel turns is to clear and cleanse my space and re-decorate it for the new festival with things I have collected on my connection walk. It is a powerful and simple ritual. I have included within each festival section some of the traditional correspondences that connect with the Celtic and Nordic spiritual traditions and folklore for decoration inspiration. To cleanse, dusting is a powerful energy shifter on its own. But if you want to do something more, you could smudge your space with sage. Or if, like me, you don't always have time to smudge and cleanse, then here is a recipe I found for a DIY cleansing all-purpose cleaning spray that is zero waste, which I use myself each festival to cleanse my altar.

DIY CLEANSING ALL-PURPOSE CLEANER[1]

Ingredients:
- Lemon rind (for joy, friendship, rejuvenation and happiness).
- Orange rind (for attracting luck).
- Thyme (for cleansing any negative energy).
- Sage (for cleansing).
- Rosemary (to uplift the energy in your home and protect).
- Distilled white vinegar.
- Distilled salt water.

How to make:
1. Put your herbs and rinds in a clean sealable glass bottle or Mason jar.
2. Cover with distilled vinegar.
3. Leave for 3–4 weeks out of the light, shake it from time to time.
4. Strain the infused vinegar.
5. Mix with some distilled salt water.
6. Put in a spray bottle and use it to clean.

FIND YOUR NATURE SPOT

Find a special space in nature. I recommend it is a quiet place where you will not be disturbed or feel as though you may be interrupted. It can be difficult when you live in the city to find such a place. However, in most parks you can find places of stillness and contemplation. Your space might change depending on your lifestyle. A person who travels much may have sacred spaces all over the world. Or it could simply be within your own garden. It needs to be a place you can visit frequently. Wherever you find it, spend time there as often as possible. Not only is this a place to connect with nature, this is also a place where you can recharge and meditate.

---

[1] Adapted from a recipe by the Cookery Witch on Youtube.

PUT THE FESTIVAL DATES IN YOUR CALENDAR

Life can speed away with us, so I highly recommend putting the festival dates in an electronic calendar that will give you a gentle reminder, until the Wheel of the Year dates becomes more familiar to you. If you can, I recommend blocking out some time on or around the festival – even if it's just an hour to take a walk and decorate your sacred space as the seasons turn. Although, particularly for the solstices and equinoxes, the seasons' shifts are strongest on the actual dates, I tend to think you can still feel that energy in the week before and week after. So, if that is when you can make time for the festival then that is okay.

**Are you ready to begin your journey?
Then walk with me as the wheel turns…………**

Samhain

31st OCTOBER

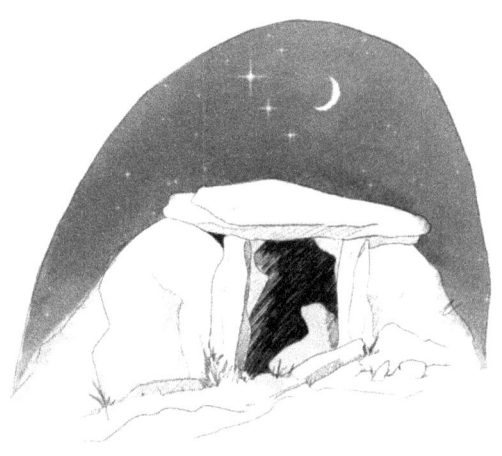

The wheel has turned once more…
As the old year dies and a new begins.
For one night the ancestors return,
Before the new wheel starts to spin…

Samhain

HONOURING THE CYCLE OF DEATH AND REBIRTH

Connecting with the season:
Before you read the chapter on Samhain in the *Walking the Wheel of the Year* book, take a walk alone outside and find a quiet place where you feel comfortable and do the Tree of Life Meditation (p. 203).

Now continue your walk. As we walk at each festival, this is a time to reflect upon nature's journey as the macrocosm, and our journey in life as the microcosm. It is a moment to bring yourself into flow with the season. As you walk, reflect upon the following questions and, when you come home to your sacred space, write down the answers to the following questions below:

> *** Remember to look for the signs of Samhain now, not the signs you would expect to be looking for. We tend to have preconceived ideas of what each season 'should' look like in nature and in our lives. There is no 'should'. And with climate change, the seasons are starting to look very different each year. To attune to nature, we have to look beyond preconceptions and see what is happening here and now. ***

P.S. For the best insight, write freely and from your heart. Nothing you write here can be wrong or right – it just needs to make sense to you. This is your moment and space to reflect.

What signs of autumn and winter can you see around you?

_____
_____
_____
_____
_____

How has the world around you changed in the last 12 months?

_____
_____
_____
_____
_____

How has your life changed in the last 12 months?

_____
_____
_____
_____
_____

Can you see a connection between your life's journey and nature's journey?

_____
_____
_____
_____
_____

> Now read Chapter 5: Samhain – Honouring the Cycle of Death and Rebirth in the *Walking the Wheel of the Year* book (pp.27–41). You can read just the history and then come back to do the following exercises, or the entire chapter and then come here to do the processes.

GROWING WITH THE SEASON

Letting go

At Samhain, we ask ourselves: what will we take with us into this new cycle? What do we choose to leave behind?

Use this space to create a representation of everything in your life that is positive, negative, and in-between. You could make a collage or drawing of yourself surrounded with keywords describing both the negative and positive influences in your life. Or, if you prefer, you could just write keywords in a table or a list. Remember to include your achievements, both the big and small things from the past wheel, as well as those things that make you happy in your life and, equally, those things that make you sad.

When you have made the representation of your life, have a good look at it. Take a step back and ask yourself:

- What becomes immediately obvious?
- Can I see the positive and negative influences within the last year?
- Importantly, can I identify the parts of my life and beliefs that are holding me back?

Contemplate the patterns presented and your observations. Now ask yourself:

- What will I take forward with me in the new wheel?
- What will I leave behind and let go of?

Circle the keywords that represent the things you want to leave behind.

Now, in your sacred space, and in a metal container, light a small candle or charcoal block. Read each statement aloud and then say, 'I banish you from my life,' then burn the paper. Thank it and let it go.

If you like, you can keep these for the transformation crafting in the *WTWOTY* book (p.30), or you can release them to the wind.

ANCESTORS

Samhain is the time of remembering our roots and where we come from. A time to honour those who gave us our gifts, our personalities, our DNA. It is a time to pay respect to those who walked the earth before us. Remember, if you know where you have come from, you have a better idea of where you are going.

Find a picture of someone in your family who has died who you feel drawn to. If you have not got someone, then instead choose an important person in your life who inspired you immensely who has passed over.

In the following space, write about them, and their life. Share a memory you have. Have a look and see how this person affected your life, and what they taught you. Put their picture in your sacred space until Yule to honour their memory and the gifts they gave you.

To deepen your connection with them, think of something you can do to honour the memory of the person you have connected with in this exercise. It could be that you visit their burial site. Alternatively, it could be that you do an activity that you used to share with this person. My favourite action is to write this person a letter as though I am talking to them, thanking them for their gifts and the role they played in my journey.

What will you do to honour this person?
Write your ideas below:

_____
_____
_____
_____
_____
_____
_____

CELEBRATING SAMHAIN

One of the most important parts of the Wheel of the Year to our ancestors was the celebration of the festivals of the wheel. Like our modern-day festivals such as Christmas, traditionally, after the ceremony, festivals were celebrated with local customs, and of course no Celtic or Nordic festival would have been complete without a feast!

However, speaking from experience, in our 21st-century lives, a feast eight times a year might not be something there is time and capacity for. But, the fantastic thing about celebrating the Wheel of the Year today is that we can make new traditions, inspired by the past, but which are more relevant to our lives today. In the *Walking the Wheel of the Year* book (pp.32–36), you will find inspiration for Samhain traditions and crafts that you could incorporate into your Samhain celebrations.

So, how will you celebrate Samhain?
Here's some space for you to write your ideas:

SYMBOLISM OF SAMHAIN

There is much traditional symbolism that corresponds to each festival. I always say that your sacred space should be decorated in a way that feels right to you. However, if you would like to have some traditional symbolism, here is a list:

Symbolism of Samhain:
Ancestors, death, rebirth, remembrance.

Symbols of Samhain:
Apples, pomegranates, fire, pumpkins, jack-a-lanterns, cauldron, photographs of deceased family and friends.

Colours:
Orange, red, yellow, brown, dark yellow, dark green, black, purple.

Foods:
Apples, pomegranates, pork, nuts, roasted game birds, cider, dark wine, pears, root vegetables.

Herbs:
Rosemary, calendula, myrrh or patchouli.

Flowers:
Calendula, chrysanthemum, wild ginseng, wormwood.

Animals:
Blackbirds, bats, cats (particularly black cats), owls, spiders, ravens.

Goddesses:
Cerridwen (Welsh), Persephone (Greek), Aradia (Italian), the Norns (Norse), Hecate (Greek), Lillith (Hebrew), death goddesses, dying and rising goddesses.

Gods:
Cernunnos (Celtic), all wine deities, Odin (Norse), the Horned God (British), Herne the Hunter (Celtic), Bran (Welsh).

CEREMONY

As I wrote in the *Walking the Wheel of the Year* book (pp.20–23), I believe that one of the most beautiful and powerful ways you can connect to the season's energy is through ceremony. However, I also strongly believe there is no right or wrong way of doing ceremony. That said, I feel it is important that ceremonies are thought about, planned and should never be done just for the sake of holding ceremony. The only exception I have to that rule is a spontaneous gratitude circle, where I simply give thanks for the gifts in my life.

Creating your own ceremony can be daunting, which is why in the *Walking the Wheel of the Year* book I have included my own seasonal ceremonies as inspiration for you. Yet, I strongly recommend you to create your own when it feels comfortable to do so.

I believe the best and most powerful ceremonies come from the heart. Therefore, in my opinion, you should never do something in a ceremony that you feel is not right for you. Ceremony doesn't need to be complicated unless you wish it to be. And above all, it should mean something and make sense only to you. It could be as simple as lighting candles and meditating or making a traditional craft. It could be the mindful act of cleansing and redecorating your altar.

And, for me, it is the mindfulness that is important. Ceremony, in my humble opinion, should be about creating a time within a time and a space within a space. In other words, creating a moment in time and space that is sacred and intimate for you to connect with yourself and with what is important to you. For me, that is always my ancestors, the elements, and the gods and goddesses I follow. For you, that will be different. As you are interested in following the wheel and a nature-based spiritual path, I would suggest inviting the five core elements of nature (Earth, Air, Fire, Water, and Spirit) into your ceremony, whether that be a formal invite into creating a traditional pagan-esque sacred circle or simply physically represented on your altar.

CEREMONY PLANNER

What is the purpose/intention of the ceremony?

Where and when will the ceremony be held?

How will I create sacred space (including how the ceremony will start and end)?

What activities will happen during the ceremony (including tools/items needed)?

Words to create sacred space/begin the ceremony[2]:

Words for activities, prayers, gratitude:

Words to end the ceremony:

---

2 It is important to really think through what you want to say in ceremony.

SAMHAIN JOURNEY

For each season in the *WTWOTY* book, there is a visualisation journey for you to try. Travelling via the World Tree, each journey connects your unconscious to the personal development themes – deepening both your connection to the seasons' energies and your personal development and growth. You can find the Samhain Journey in the *Walking the Wheel of the Year* book (p.37).

When you have completed your journey, as you slowly recover, write down or draw what you can remember from your journey (as I always say, recovering includes drinking water and eating some good chocolate!). Your journey may not make sense to you now, but it will one day.

_____

_____

_____

_____

_____

_____

_____

_____

_____

_____

_____

_____

_____

_____

_____

_____

_____

AS THE WHEEL TURNS...

Of all the festivals, Samhain is really the festival of reconnecting with your roots. If you want to deepen your root connection between Samhain and Yule, then you can continue your rooting journey. Rooting is truly about learning about the foundations of who you are and honouring them.

Whoever you were in the past has created the person you are today. Rooting can be challenging and bring up a lot of emotions. Please be kind to yourself if you choose to go in deep, and remember this is not about judging – it is about accepting and honouring. Nature doesn't judge. She just is. She evolves, adapts to her surroundings, and grows. In a way, think of rooting as a grounding and as a celebration of the journey you have taken.

If these activities bring up something challenging, then please seek professional support. We are not designed to do everything alone.

Here's some inspiration for rooting activities you can incorporate into your life until Yule. Remember, you don't have to do all of this. Do what makes sense for you and your life.

- Practice the Tree of Life meditation once a week.
- Visit family and friends.
- Look through old photographs and reflect upon where you came from.
- Free-write in a journal about your roots and your reflections.
- Research family history.
- Visit ancient sites or woodlands.
- Revisit activities you used to enjoy to see what they bring to you.

I wish you a magical and merry Samhain!
Blessings,

Emma-Jane xxxx

YOUR NOTES

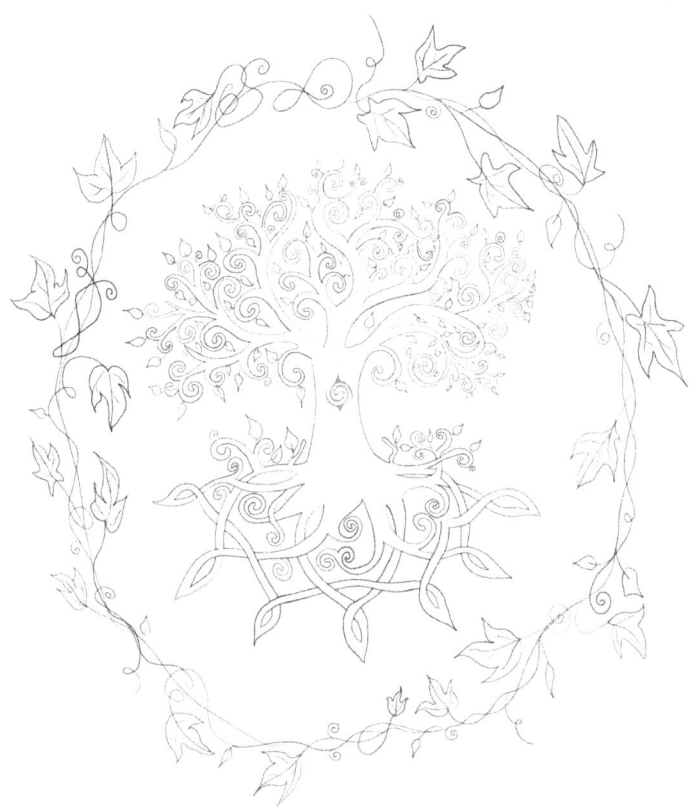

Yule and the Winter Solstice

20th/21st/22nd DECEMBER

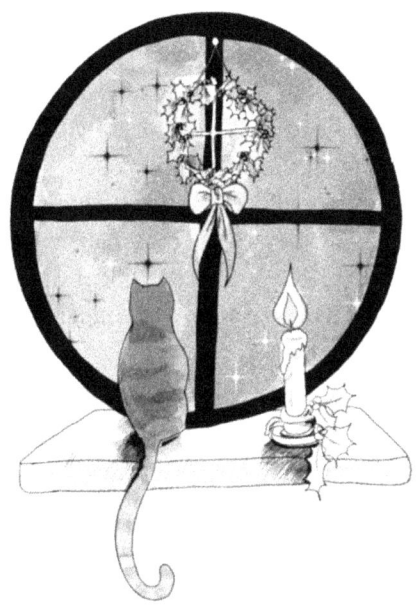

The wheel has turned once more…
Through the longest night the sun is born.
A time to gather around the hearth,
A time to feast and to laugh…

Yule

HONOURING THE CYCLE OF DEATH AND REBIRTH

Connecting with the season

The wheel has turned and it is time to reflect and feel into the energy of Yule, the winter solstice. Before you read the chapter on Yule in the *Walking the Wheel of the Year* book, take a walk alone outside and find a quiet place where you feel comfortable and do the Tree of Life Meditation (p.203).

Now continue your walk. Remember that this is a time to reflect upon nature's journey as the macrocosm, and our journey in life as the microcosm. As you walk, reflect upon the following questions. When you come home to your sacred space, write down the answers.

> *** You could combine your Yule connection walk with bringing in the green, particularly if you intend to create a Yule sunwheel (*WTWOTY* book, pp.53–54). This is a time-honoured tradition at Yule and you can read about it in the *WTWOTY* book (p.48). ***

P.S. Before the solar festivals on the Wheel of the Year, you may find that your life goes a bit wobbly (for want of a better word). Then, after the solstice, things begin to calm down. It can be interesting to do a connection walk pre and post solstice to notice and connect with the energy shifts.

What signs of winter do you see? How has the world around you changed since Samhain?

_____
_____
_____
_____
_____

How has your life changed since Samhain/summer solstice?

_____
_____
_____
_____
_____

How is this season's energy reflecting where you are in your life right now?

_____
_____
_____
_____
_____

> Now read Chapter 6: Yule and the Winter Solstice – Honouring the Gifts and Joy in Life, in *Walking the Wheel of the Year* (pp.42–60). You can read just the history and then come back to do the following exercises, or the entire chapter and then turn to this workbook to do the processes.

GROWING WITH THE SEASON

The gifts in our Lives

At Samhain, we honoured those that have passed on. Yule, however, has been, and still is, a time of celebrating the people in our lives that we love – particularly by giving gifts. The people we love bring gifts into our lives – gifts that cannot be wrapped and often don't get noticed. If we take the premise that every person in our life is a teacher and has something to share with us, and we with them, then we can learn so much. By consciously looking at the gifts the people we love give to us, we can begin to identify not only why people are important to us but also why we needed to learn the teachings their gifts brought – shedding a new light on bits of yourself you may not have seen clearly before.

Look at the people on your gift list. Choose one or two people and, on the following page, ask yourself:

- Who are these people?
- What is their relationship to you?
- What gifts have they brought to your life (this can be stability, lessons, love)?
- For each gift, think about your life and why this teaching is necessary to your life today.

> **Bonus activities: Thanking your community**
> Write these people letters thanking them for the gifts they bring to your life. And if possible, spend time with them, get to know them on a deeper level and reflect more upon the gifts they bring to your life.

FINDING YOUR GIFTS

Gifts do not only travel one way. As we receive from people in our lives, we also give them gifts and teachings, both consciously and unconsciously. It can often be a challenge to recognise the strength and inspiration we bring to others' lives. However, your gifts are as unique as you are and they light up the world in their own way. Yule is a wonderful time to recognise how you bring light to the world.

Ask yourself:

- What gifts do you give to others?
- What do people come to you for help with?

Use the empty space below to write down your gifts:

Now, choose the three that you feel most proud of this Yule and, on the next page, in each candle, write these three gifts that you give to people and the world.

THE GIFTS I BRING TO THE WORLD

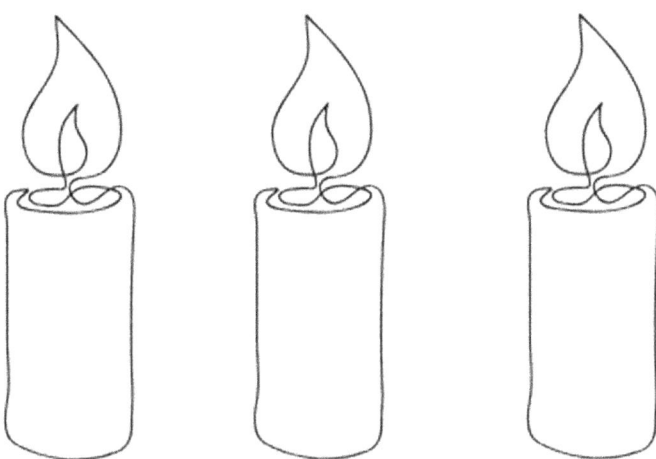

> *** **Inspiration** ***
> You could place three candles in your sacred space to represent these gifts. As a way of honouring my gifts, I like to incorporate the following activity into my Yule ceremony. I light my three candles one at a time. As I do this, I say out loud:
> 'I bring the gift of .... to the world.
> I am grateful that I can share this gift with the world.'

CONNECTING WITH YOUR INNER CHILD

The phrase 'connecting with your inner child' can conjure up the image of old wounds buried deeply in our psyche, creating the belief that inner child work is a serious business and an area for deep healing (and, on one level, yes it absolutely is). However, our inner child is also that part of us that represents our capacity for innocence, wonder, awe, joy, sensitivity and playfulness – and Yule energy is abundant with the exact same energy. Working joyfully with your inner child at this time of year is seasonally perfect as, of course, Yule is the time of the birth of the summer sun. By connecting with our childlike energy joyfully and allowing our inner child to appreciate this time of year, we can connect with a magic in our lives that we don't often give ourselves time or permission to during the rest of the year.

There are many, many ways to connect with your inner child, but the most powerful will always be through play and activities that we loved as children, particularly through stories. At Yule, our ancestors used to tell stories on the longest night – and a great way to learn more about yourself and reconnect with your inner child is to revisit the stories of your childhood. So, what could be more appropriate at Yule than returning to those stories?

CHILDHOOD STORIES

Think back to the stories you loved as a child, the stories that have stayed with you.

Choose the one that is most memorable to you right now. If possible, tell someone the story as you remember it (not as it was written), or write it briefly below.

Story Name:

_____

_____

Now reflect on these following questions:

What did this story teach you?

_____
_____
_____
_____

Did this lesson stay with you throughout your life, or for just a period of your life?

_____
_____
_____
_____

Has the lesson changed from when you were a child to now as an adult?

_____
_____
_____
_____

Which story would you pass on to another generation and why?

_____
_____
_____
_____

> Throughout this wheel, return to your story and see if the meaning changes for you. This is a great exercise to do every Yule, as different stories are apparent at different times. The story you tell this Yule might not be the same story you tell next Yule …

INNER CHILD PLAYDATE

Children have a unique worldview and live in the present, which we as adults forget. Allowing yourself to play as an adult can be challenging. We have a social construct that tells us that when we become an adult, we need to be serious. Yet, play is just as important for adults as it is for children. It's vital for problem-solving, creativity and relationships. Play makes us more innovative. Think how a child's mind works. In their imagination, they can turn sand into a cake made of ice cream and sausages, or blankets into magical flying capes, and houses into castles. They embrace infinite possibilities without question and ignore the limitations of reality. To a child, a plastic doll is a living, breathing being. As adults, it can be challenging to get immediately into this place of imagination. Which is why connecting with your inner child tangibly through play is so important in helping you to engage a child's world, imagination and joy. Yule is the perfect time to set some valuable time aside for an inner child playdate.

There are many, many ways to have an inner child playdate. Here are some ideas for you to try.

Find your joy – Think about what it was you used to love about this time of year as a child. Spend a day or an afternoon doing things you loved, or the things you always wished you could do at this time of year but never got to do, and find that joy.

Build a pillow fort! – One of the best ways to connect with your inner child is to build a pillow fort, as this will not only be a natural connection with play but also a seasonal hibernation space for you mentally and physically!

Take a 'wonder' wander – If you have ever been for a walk with a small child, you know that it takes a long time. Children love to notice and explore the world around them. And what is stopping us from doing the same? Get yourself outside and allow yourself to marvel at the world around you. The sparkling lights, the frost in the air, watching people laugh and love each other. When we stop to notice, this world is full of so many magical moments we can enjoy.

Demonstrate kindness – Children are naturally filled with love and a desire to be kind to one another. They hug and kiss the things and people they love without question. Actively and demonstrably practicing gratitude is a great way to connect with our inner child's ability to love implicitly. Doing actions of love and kindness for others is a great way to really allow your inner child to come out. Write a letter of thanks for one you love, give a gift to a coworker who has helped you this year, donate food to a food bank and, if you are able, volunteer and give your time to help people who are alone at this time of year. Caring for the world in childlike compassion will allow you to feel love in its purest form.

Remember to laugh! – Laughter awakens the inner child from his or her slumber. So, allow yourself to be silly and laugh this Yule. Silly games, comedy films, and even attacking those perfect Yuletide crafts and recipes from TikTok with the enthusiasm and confidence of a five-year-old will bring a smile to your lips and to your inner child's heart!

CELEBRATING YULE

Yule can be a challenge to celebrate, as roughly 80% of us are celebrating Christmas with family and friends, and it can all get a bit hectic to try and celebrate Yule. Living in an international household, where one person is very dedicated to a spiritual life and the other is not on a specific spiritual path but, however, loves a traditional Christmas, I often get asked how we do it. Well, the great thing about Yule is that a lot of the modern-day traditions come from our ancestors Yule traditions, so we have adapted to incorporate what is meaningful to us. When we go out for our Christmas tree, we bring in the green, make a sun wheel, and then burn a Yule log with some of last year's green upon it. We celebrate with a Yule feast on the longest night, Danish Christmas (24th December), and British Christmas (25th December). I like to think that my Celtic ancestors would approve of the many days of good food, as they really loved to feast. And, personally, I observe the sunrises and sunsets over the three days of the solstice (the day before, of, and after), and I do the very exercises that you have been doing here – either before Yule over the month or after, as time allows. My inner child playdate is often part of the recovery (post-Christmas guests process, for example).

Remember that in celebrating the Wheel of the Year today, we can make new traditions inspired by the past but which are more relevant to our lives today. In the *Walking the Wheel of the Year* book (pp.48–55), you will find inspiration for Yule traditions and crafts that you could incorporate into your own celebrations.

So, how will you celebrate Yule?
Here's some space for you to write your ideas:

SYMBOLISM OF YULE

Rebirth, childhood, inner child, gratitude, joy, misrule, survival, growth.

Symbols of Yule:

Yule tree, sun wheel, holly & ivy, candles, Yule wreaths, feasting, Yule log.

Colours:

Gold, green, red, white, silver.

Foods:

Apple cider, cinnamon cakes, oranges, dried fruits, eggnog, gingerbread, mulled wine, roasted and spiced meats, roasted apples, nut loaf, the Wassail cup, mead, cranberries.

Herbs:

Cinnamon, ginger, dried chamomile flowers, juniper berries, peppermint, nutmeg.

Flowers and trees:

Holly, oak, mistletoe, ivy, evergreens, laurel, bayberry, blessed thistle, frankincense, pine, sage, yellow cedar, ash (for the Yule log).

Animals:

Bears, deer, owls, phoenix, reindeer, snow geese, squirrels, stags, robins.

Goddesses:

Frigga (Norse), Cailleach Bheur (Celtic), Frau Holle (Norse), La Befana (Italian), Mother Earth.

Gods:

Baldur (Norse), the Horned God (British), trickster gods, Herne the Hunter (Celtic), the Oak King and the Holly King.

CEREMONY PLANNER

What is the purpose/intention of the ceremony?

Where and when will the ceremony be held?

How will I create sacred space (including how the ceremony will start and end)?

What activities will happen during the ceremony (including tools/items needed)?

Words to create sacred space/begin the ceremony:[3]

Words for activities, prayers, gratitude:

Words to end the ceremony:

---

3 It is important to really think through what you want to say in ceremony.

YULE JOURNEY

You can find the Yule Journey in the *Walking the Wheel of the Year* book (pp.56–57). Once you have done your journey, as you slowly recover, write down or draw what you can remember from your journey (remember that recovering includes drinking water and eating some good chocolate!).

AS THE WHEEL TURNS...

Post-Yule, the sun's new light and energy brings us inspiration, new dreams and plans – often expressed in January by New Year's resolutions. However, when walking the wheel, we first begin to act upon these ideas in the early spring at Imbolc. From Yule to Imbolc in February, this is still a time of hibernation that is truly important to both creating sustainable steps forward in your life and living a life that flows with nature's rhythm, not against it.

Growth within nature is slower, gradual, almost unnoticeable. By hibernating and allowing natural inspiration, plans and visions become clearer, sharper. In the Wheel of the Year, we begin to grow our goals at Imbolc. However, in order to put new goals and dreams into action, we need to first collect our inspiration.

Here is some inspiration for different activities you can incorporate into your life until Imbolc. As always, these are for inspiration only – do what makes sense for you and your life.

- Keep an inspiration diary of ideas for your upcoming goals and projects for the rest of the wheel.
- Practice the Tree of Life Meditation once a week.
- Allow yourself to hibernate a little and start the year slowly.
- Collect images or phrases that you can use for your Imbolc vision board.
- Have another playdate with your inner child.
- Leave out food for birds that may be struggling to find food this time of year.

I wish you a magical and merry Yule!
Blessings,

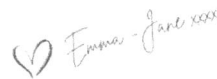

YOUR NOTES

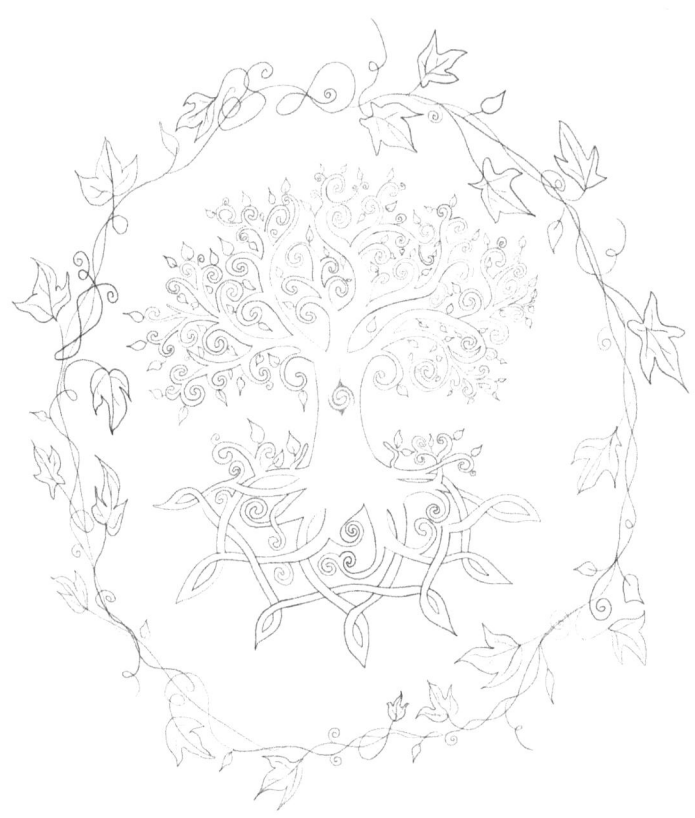

Imbolc

2nd FEBRUARY

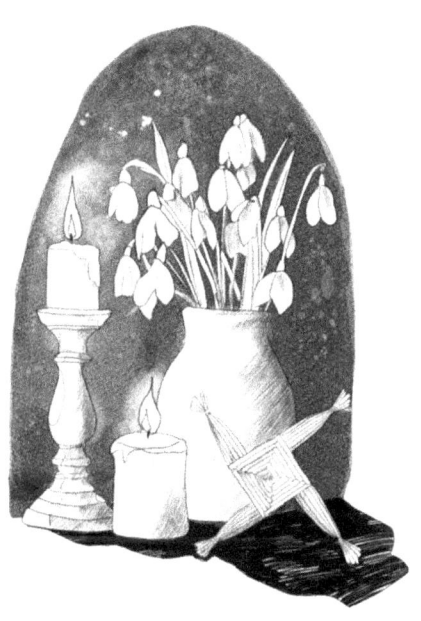

The wheel has turned once more…
The land begins to stir.
As bud and shoot and leaf unfurls,
Inspiration fills the air…

Imbolc

INFINITE NEW BEGINNINGS AND POSSIBILITIES

Connecting with the season

The wheel has turned to Imbolc. The air is warmer with a hint of frost, and the snow has melted away, leaving the land beneath rich and fertile. Although the air is frosty, colour is subtly beginning to come back to the land, pale and misty. The buds are gently starting to show hints of opening, small shoots carefully poke their tips above the earth. Gently, the land is awakening. Spring bubbles beneath the land. New life is coming – what will it bring?

Before you read the chapter on Imbolc in the *Walking the Wheel of the Year* book, take a walk alone outside and find a quiet place where you feel comfortable and do the Tree of Life Meditation (p.203).

Now continue your walk. Remember, this is a time to reflect upon nature's journey as the macrocosm, and our journey in life as the microcosm. As you walk, reflect upon the following questions, and when you come home to your sacred space, write down the answers.

How has the world around you changed since Yule?

_____
_____
_____
_____
_____

How has your life changed since Yule?

_____
_____
_____
_____
_____

Can you see the connections between nature's changes and your life's changes?

_____
_____
_____
_____
_____

How is this season's energy reflecting where you are in your life right now?

_____
_____
_____
_____
_____

> Now read Chapter 7: Imbolc – Infinite New Beginnings and Possibilities, in the *Walking the Wheel of the Year* book (pp.61–63).
> You can read just the history and then come back to do the following exercises, or the entire chapter and then come to this workbook to do the processes.

GROWING WITH THE SEASON

Clarifying the vision

The dreaming hibernation time from Yule to Imbolc and the newly growing light give us inspiration and energy. At Imbolc, we begin the process of setting goals to manifest throughout this wheel, just as our ancestors planned their crops. Which means this is the time to clarify your vision for your goals, the crops you will plant in your life during this wheel. The important questions to ask yourself here are: how do I want my life to be? What do I actually want to manifest?

This process can seem quite daunting. However, inspiration comes from the strangest of places – both positive and negative. Personally, I find that after Yule I often hit a low point in both my energy and motivation. Sometimes I become dissatisfied with my current position in my life. Although this may sound negative, these emotions can actually be used to inspire change. They show us that something in our lives is not ok. Something needs to change.

I like to think of these feelings as a gift, a hidden teaching. When we choose to look at why we are feeling a particular way, and by using these negative feelings to inspire us, we take control of our lives and become powerful. So, if you have any negativity or low energy at the moment, look into it.

On the flip side, joy is a huge inspiration factor for changing your life or manifesting goals. After all, who doesn't want to feel happy and joyful in life?! If you have been spending time with your inner child since Yule, then you will (hopefully) have remembered the joy of play and what really makes you happy at your core and centre. Your inner child or your unconscious can often, if not always, be your very best guide to truly being happy in life.

Use the following questions to truly ask yourself how you want your life to be. Allow yourself to write freely and rapidly. Sometimes, setting a timer is a great way to stop the over-thinking that distracts our adult brain. Don't bother with unimportant things like spelling and grammar right now. Just as long as you understand it, that's all that matters.

What am I unsatisfied with/unhappy about in my life at the moment (go on, have a good moan!)?

_____
_____
_____
_____
_____

What do these feelings tell me about how my life needs to change?

_____
_____
_____
_____
_____

What do I love to do that makes me forget time, food and bathroom breaks?

_____
_____
_____
_____
_____

How did I like to spend my time as a child?

_____
_____
_____
_____

If I had to leave the house every day, and only return to eat and sleep, what would I do with my time that would fulfill me?

_____
_____
_____
_____
_____

What drains me?

_____
_____
_____
_____
_____

What energizes me?

_____
_____
_____
_____
_____

If I could only manifest one thing, what would be the thing that would make the biggest impact on my life and bring me the most joy?

_____
_____
_____
_____
_____

PLANNING YOUR GOALS

Before you do anything else, please take a seat and give yourself a big round of applause because that kind of work is not easy and you have just gone deep, fast. You may want to take a step back for 24 hours and continue this next step later.

If you're ready, let's get to my favourite bit of Imbolc – creating your goals.

First, check in. You may feel overly motivated during this time of year. After all, birth energy is explosive and intense. Often I find that millions of ideas and good intentions surface. However, to create a life you love, a sustainable life you love, you need to work gradually, to take baby steps and, of course, enjoy that journey – which is why the manifestation process I have created with the Wheel of the Year is slow and steady and happens over all the festivals.

Now please don't get me wrong when I talk about goal-setting. Life itself cannot exactly be a goal in the classic 'reach-your-target,' measurable way. Life is a journey that evolves continuously. Contentment in your life journey and a feeling of fulfilling your life are the goals we work towards whilst walking the Wheel of the Year. Just as we attune to nature's flow, we also need to mirror that by connecting with the ebbs and flows of our life's journey. We do this actively, not passively – which is why we set goals that will make slow and steady changes which will nurture your growth, soul-attunement and create joy sustainably throughout your life.

Having a clear target helps us to create a guide to navigating our journey – hence goals. Now you have some clarity about what you would like to manifest. On the next page, start by creating four to six goals that you would like to manifest by Samhain (31st October). It doesn't matter if you don't know how you manifest them yet; just having a vague idea is fine. It may be that you have had a particular goal running over a few years, such as writing a book. Writing a book is a BIG goal and you may need two or three cycles to finish it. However, for now, don't get caught in the details. If you want to make that a focus of this wheel then you can write it down.

MY GOALS

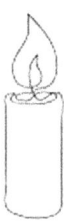

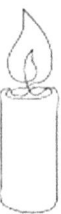

WALKING THE WHEEL OF THE YEAR COMPANION WORKBOOK

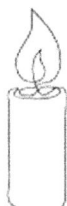

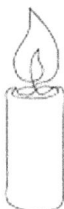

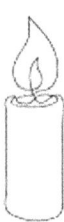

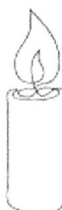

VISION BOARD

Now you are going to make a vision board to really get clear on what it is that you want to change or create. Collect images that help you visualise your four to six goals and, on a large sheet of paper, begin to paste these images around a picture of you in the centre. The picture of yourself is simply to remind you that your journey is about you. This is your wheel's vision. From now until Ostara, you will test out these ideas.

Your vision board is your personal visual reminder of your dreams. There is no right or wrong way to create it and if, like me, you choose to do this every wheel, then you will build your own method of creating your vision boards. Personally, I group my images around the picture of me – rather like a mind map.

Have fun with this activity. As children, we played with paper and glue, cutting and sticking, enjoying the simple pleasure of creating. There is no unspoken rule which says that all adult experiences should be serious. So, break out the scissors, glitter, glue, and felt tips (these may be hidden somewhere in your child's bedroom), and enjoy!

Hang your vision board in a place where you can see it every day. I have mine on the front door so I can be reminded of my intentions for the year every time I see my vision.

A little bit of candle magic

Candle magic is a very old practice that we today can align with manifestation. At Imbolc, it is traditional to make candles. You could use the following process to strengthen your manifestation vision for this year by doing a little candle magic, if that appeals to you!

MAKING CANDLES

You will need (to make four candles):

- 2 beeswax sheets.
- Wick – enough length to make the number of candles (the same height as the edge on your wax sheet plus 5cm).

How to make your candles:

1. Place a wax sheet on a cutting mat and, using a sharp knife, make a diagonal cut (you can also cut it into two rectangles).
2. If the wax is very brittle, warm it gently with a hairdryer to make it soft and pliable if necessary.
3. Lay the wick along the edge of the beeswax sheet.
4. Carefully fold the edge over the wick. Leave 5cm of the wick uncovered at the lighting end of the candle.
5. Applying even pressure with both hands, begin to roll the candle around the wick, making sure to keep it even so the bottom of the candle will be flat when it is completely rolled.

> *** **Candle magic** ***
>
> Traditional folklore candle magic is in its essence very mundane, but also very powerful. It often includes making something and focusing – like visualisation today.
>
> Whilst making your candles, focus upon your intentions for the coming wheel. Imagine that all your goals are fulfilled and achieved. Focus on how good that will feel. Keep the image of the desired result you want in complete focus.
>
> In the coming months, as you work on your goals and feel in need of inspiration, you can light your candles to connect with the Imbolc inspiration energy to help you keep going.

CELEBRATING IMBOLC

Contrasting with Yule, celebrating Imbolc, I always find, is very much a solitary journey. It is a time of looking inwards, lighting the spark of inspiration and creativity we all have in us. Yet, as Imbolc is the second of the Celtic festivals on the wheel, there are also many folk traditions and crafts that can be used to inspire a solitary or more community-based celebration.

In the *Walking the Wheel of the Year* book (pp.66–73), you will find inspiration for Imbolc traditions and crafts that you could incorporate into your Imbolc celebrations.

So, how will you celebrate Yule?

Here's some space for you to write your ideas:

SYMBOLISM OF IMBOLC:

New beginnings, inspiration, new projects, creativity, fertility, the returning light, weather magic, sacred wells.

Date of Imbolc:
Imbolc is celebrated on the 1st or 2nd of February.

Symbols of Imbolc:
Candles, milk, fire, snowdrops, Brigid's bed and doll, Brigid cross, seeds.

Colours:
White, light green, yellow, gold.

Foods:
Soups, breads, winter vegetables, seeds, milk, wine, bannocks, butter.

Herbs:
Chamomile tea, basil.

Flowers:
Snowdrops, aconite.

Animals:
Swans, ewes or sheep.

Goddesses:
Blodeuwedd, Boann, Brigid, Brighid, Bridget, Bride, Cailleach, Minerva, all virgin/maiden goddesses.

Gods:
Gods of love and fertility, Eros, Aengus, Februus, Pan, Faunus, Bragi.

CEREMONY PLANNER

What is the purpose/intention of the ceremony?

Where and when will the ceremony be held?

How will I create sacred space (including how the ceremony will start and end)?

What activities will happen during the ceremony (including tools/items needed)?

Words to create sacred space/begin the ceremony[4]:

Words for activities, prayers, gratitude:

Words to end the ceremony:

---

4 It is important to really think through what you want to say in ceremony.

IMBOLC JOURNEY

You can find the Imbolc Journey in *WTWOTY* (pp.73–74). When you have done your journey, as you slowly recover, write down or draw what you can remember from your journey (remember that recovering includes drinking water and eating some good chocolate!).

AS THE WHEEL TURNS...

The time between Imbolc and Ostara is, in my opinion at least, truly special. Surrounded by birth, growth, and light as the spring becomes more apparent, life seems to speed up. People climb out of their cosy hibernation and begin to reach out. With all this new life energy, I have noticed that people just starting to attune to the Wheel of the Year sometimes experience either a complete overwhelming or, alternatively, a try-to-do-everything and hustle attitude at this time of year. Neither is optimal. All of us walking this path have experienced this. I and others who have walked many wheels find that the easiest way to flow with this contrast in winter and spring energies is by thinking of it as surfing. Allow yourself to flow with the wave of energy as it ebbs and flows, then relax in between. You don't have to do everything. Do what feels right for you, follow your gut, and keep checking in with yourself. Most importantly, by recharging your batteries with sunlight as much as possible, you will find it much easier to flow with the spring.

Here is some inspiration for different activities you can incorporate into your life until Imbolc. As always, these are simply for inspiration. Do what makes sense for you and your life.

- Get as much sunlight as you can.
- Practice the Tree of Life Meditation once a week.
- If you have the opportunity, visit a spring or a sacred well.
- Unleash your creativity by investing some time in it. Creating can be anything, not just traditional art or poetry – making Lego is still a form of creating.
- Begin to try out some of your goals (slowly).

I wish you magical and inspiring Imbolc!
Blessings,

Emma-Jane xxxx

YOUR NOTES

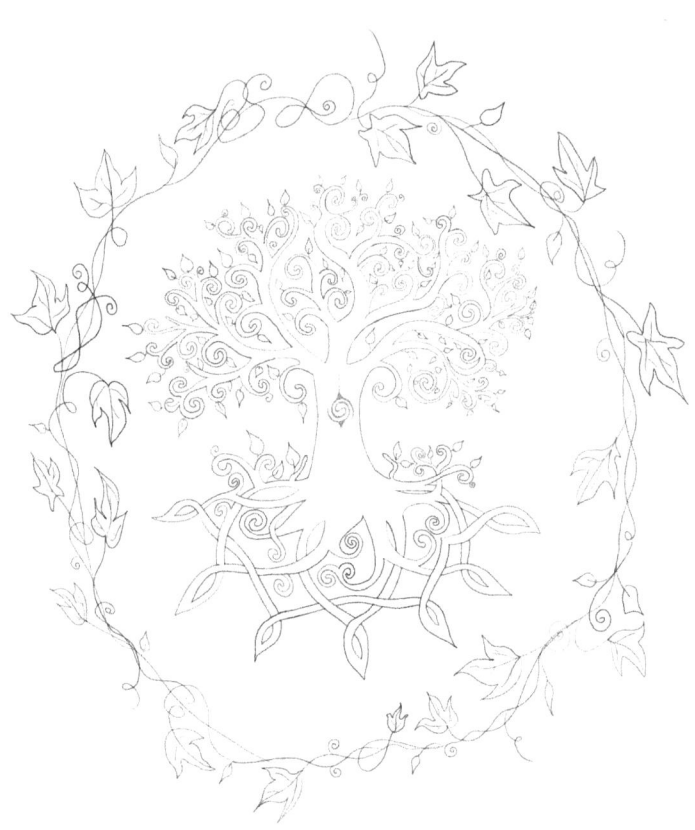

Ostara and the Spring Equinox

20th/21st/22nd DECEMBER

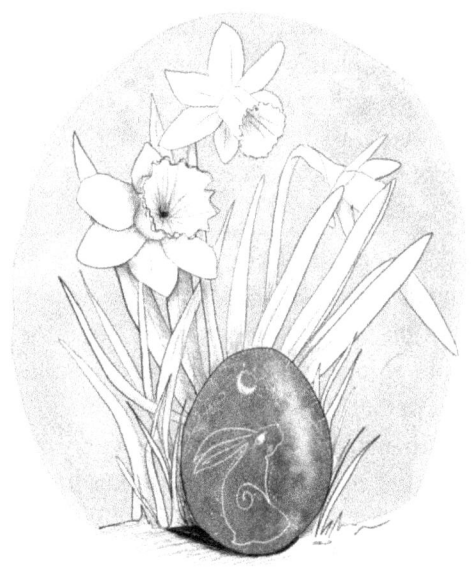

The wheel has turned once more…
Young animals enter the world.
A point of balance between light and dark,
We prepare the land and begin our work.

Ostara

CONNECTING WITH THE SEASON

The wheel has turned and it is time to reflect and feel into the energy of Ostara, the spring equinox. Before you read the chapter on Ostara in the *Walking the Wheel of the Year* book, take a walk alone outside and find a quiet place where you feel comfortable and do the Tree of Life Meditation (p.203).

Now continue your walk. Remember that this is a time to reflect upon nature's journey as the macrocosm, and our journey in life as the microcosm. As you walk, reflect upon the following questions, and when you come home to your sacred space, write down the answers.

> *** Ostara is the second of the solar festivals on the Wheel of the Year and, as with all solar festivals, you may find that your life goes a bit wobbly (for want of a better word), and then afterwards things begin to calm down. I was always taught that, particularly with the solar festivals, it is powerful and insightful to observe the energy over three days. The day before, the day of, and the day after. I find that it really helps me to tune into and flow with the 'wobbly energy' and transition to rootedness post-solar festival. ***

How has the world around you changed since Imbolc?
_____
_____
_____
_____
_____

How has your life changed since Imbolc and Yule?

_____
_____
_____
_____
_____

Can you see the connections between nature's changes and your life's changes?

_____
_____
_____
_____
_____

How is this season's energy reflecting where you are in your life right now?

_____
_____
_____
_____
_____

> Now read Chapter 8: Ostara and the Spring Equinox – Birth and Balance, in the *Walking the Wheel of the Year* book (pp.77–98).
>
> You can read just the history and then come back to do the following exercises, or the entire chapter and then come to this workbook to do the processes.

GROWING WITH THE SEASON

Taking action to manifest goals
Spring cleaning
It might seem a strange place to start – with a clearing. However, it is in fact bringing us home into the wheel's rhythm. Farmers have to clear the fields before planting seeds, after all.

Every new piece of work takes some clearing and preparation to begin. We need to clear out the dirt, dust and debris of winter to make room for the new growth that we are creating within our lives. Additionally, I find that when we tidy around ourselves, we also tidy within ourselves.

So grab a duster, chuck out the old bills you have no use for and, if you want a good cleansing after all that hard work, then book yourself in for a spa day. After all, cleaning doesn't have to be all hard work!

Evaluating your goals
Since Imbolc, you (hopefully) have been beginning to try out your new projects. From this, you will see if you have created a manageable goal or not.

Sometimes we can set ourselves up for a fail by trying to do too much too fast. Don't worry if you have – we all do this (I am known for doing this if I don't keep myself in check!).

Look again at your vision boards. Ask yourself:

- What projects have started to work?
- Have any projects been challenging to begin?
- Have you forgotten any of your dreams?
- Which projects have been flowing naturally?
- Have you had any success so far, or are you finding it difficult to focus and create the visions you set for yourself?

On the next pages, analyse the goals you set at Imbolc and modify them if you feel they are unrealistic for this wheel.

Goal 1:

What has worked?

_____
_____
_____

What hasn't worked?

_____
_____
_____

Why hasn't it worked so far?

_____
_____
_____

What can you do differently to make it work?

_____
_____
_____

Redefined/New goal:

_____
_____
_____

Goal 2:

What has worked?
_____
_____
_____

What hasn't worked?
_____
_____
_____

Why hasn't it worked so far?
_____
_____
_____

What can you do differently to make it work?
_____
_____
_____

Redefined/New goal:
_____
_____
_____

Goal 3:

What has worked?
_____
_____
_____

What hasn't worked?

_____

_____

Why hasn't it worked so far?

_____

_____

_____

What can you do differently to make it work?

_____

_____

_____

Redefined/New goal:

_____

_____

_____

Goal 4:

What has worked?

_____

_____

What hasn't worked?

_____

_____

_____

Why hasn't it worked so far?

_____

_____

_____

What can you do differently to make it work?
_____
_____
_____

Redefined/New goal:
_____
_____
_____

Goal 5:

What has worked?
_____
_____
_____

What hasn't worked?
_____
_____
_____

Why hasn't it worked so far?
_____
_____
_____

What can you do differently to make it work?
_____
_____
_____

Redefined/New goal:
_____
_____
_____

Goal 6:

What has worked?
_____
_____

What hasn't worked?
_____
_____

Why hasn't it worked so far?
_____
_____

What can you do differently to make it work?
_____
_____

Redefined/New goal:
_____
_____

Believing and doing

When manifesting goals, it is sometimes easy to allow our negative internal dialogue to not believe that we can do it, especially if we have struggled to manifest in the past. You need to rewire the brain for belief, to challenge all of your falsely constructed beliefs about your lack of ability to change your life. The Ostara teaching is simply about getting on with it anyway, despite the hurdles you have to overcome. Our ancestors had huge hurdles to overcome, inventing farming with stone and antler tools, but they did it anyway – and today we have bread.

Using visualisation techniques or positive self-talk can be really helpful to rewire the brain to believe in yourself. No matter how small or limited you believe your abilities to be, there will have been times in your life where you have succeeded in manifesting things you wanted. For example, you may have wanted to be on a specific education course or get a particular job – and you did. How? By you dreaming it and making it happen by applying and passing the interviews. You wanted to date a specific person, so you were brave and asked them. Do you see what I mean? It can be helpful to look at these accomplishments to remind you how powerful you really are. Below, write a list of things you have actively manifested in your life, to show yourself how amazing you really are:

_____
_____
_____
_____
_____
_____
_____
_____
_____

Planning

The MOST IMPORTANT step towards manifesting your goals is planning the actions that you will take.

Now it's time to translate all your dreams into practical actions, to make your plan and follow it. Step by step.

The guidelines for the actions you will take will keep you earthed and rooted on your journey, as well as nourish your motivation. Ultimately, to succeed, remember to keep your plans simple, practical and achievable. For each of your goals, you need to brainstorm/plan the dedicated actions you will take to manifest it. This makes it easy to measure your progress and keep on track.

This can be easier with practical goals such as planning a holiday, and more difficult with abstract goals like developing confidence. The key here is to really focus on action. What can you do? I always say, 'The gods help those that help themselves.'

On the blank notes pages, brainstorm ideas for action steps and then, once you are clear, write your plans on the following pages.

*** Whilst making your action plans, bear in mind that you are aiming to manifest your goals by Samhain, 31st October. So, be realistic. Your goals are to enhance your life, not overwhelm you. Be aware that some goals you will work on more and some less – thus is the ebb and flow of life. Think of these action plans as guidelines for the next few months and use them to focus on your goals. For all of the remaining festivals, we will check in on your progress and tweak these plans where it is needed. Just as the farmers tend their crops until harvest time. ***

Goal:

Action steps:

-
-
-
-

Goal:

Action steps:

-
-
-
-

Goal:

Action steps:

-
-
-
-

Goal:

Action steps:

-
-
-
-

Goal:

Action steps:
-
-
-
-

Goal:

Action steps:
-
-
-
-

Starting

Like a farmer planning his crops, you know what you want. You have done the preparation. So, now it is just time to get on with it. Begin following your actions plans.

Aim to work on one of your goals each day or each week. Once you have completed a step, check it off on your plan and move forward. Keep a note of your progress, mentally or physically.

Visualisation tool for manifestation

Visualisation is one of the most powerful processes to support goal manifestation. Visualisation at its essence is a 'mental rehearsal'. It is the process of creating a mental image or intention of what you want to happen or feel in reality.

Visualisation works best as a daily practice to support the actions you are going to take to manifest your goals. You can choose to visualise the outcome of achieving your goal, or you can choose to visualise the positive outcome action you will take that day.

How to visualise what you want:

- Close your eyes and think of the goal.
- Concentrate on the image of the positive outcome of your goal, not the steps you will have to take.
- Take several deep breaths.
- Visualize the object, the situation or result that you desire in your mind as clearly and with as much detail as you can (you can choose to visualise the steps to getting there but, personally, I prefer to focus on the result and allow my actions and the universe to figure out the how).
- Add emotion, feeling, and your senses to your vision. Feel the happiness, imagine the heat on the beach, etc.
- Hold the vision for 2–5 minutes.

SHADOW SELF

Equinox symbolically represents the balancing point between two energies. Spring equinox transitions us from the darker side of the year to the lighter, from the shadow of winter to the light of summer. The shadow is something that people often shy away from. Darkness is often viewed as something negative. Yet, when you look at it, all life, it all begins in darkness – whether in the womb or in the ground. And, as we are part of nature, we have both light and darkness within us. This is sometimes known as the shadow self and the light or higher self.

As equinoxes are the time between time, a balancing point before a transition, they remind us of the need for balance in our lives. In order to have balance in our lives and, most importantly, within ourselves, we have to accept our entire self. So, as all birth comes from darkness, here at Ostara we work with understanding and integrating our shadow self.

Our shadows are our deepest, darkest, secrets, and our deepest fears. Yet, there is strength to be found in these dark places. To understand our shadow is to understand ourselves.

However, this takes work, patience, and bravery. You have to be brave to face your shadow, and you need patience, as this part of your journey will take and should take time. You cannot do it all at once, not in one wheel. It is important to remember that the work of accepting and integrating your shadow self is by no means an easy or quick process. It is an ongoing journey. Which, if you undertake it, needs to be done with kindness, love and, wherever possible, with support.

This journey honestly sounds more daunting than it is. Do this work gently and be aware that integrating your shadow self is, at its essence, a process of embracing the shadow self – which, ultimately, is to embrace that you are perfectly imperfect and that is your strength, not your weakness.

You may feel like you don't want to do this work every wheel, and that is completely fine. You walk the wheel at your own pace. However, I would recommend always doing some form of balance work at an equinox, such as rebalancing your chakras.

EMBRACING YOUR SHADOW SELF

Identify your shadow self

The Mindfulness Solution[5] provides a simple exercise to begin to identify your shadow self:

Step 1:
Make a list of five positive qualities that you see yourself as having (e.g., compassionate, generous, witty, etc.):
-
-
-
-
-

Step 2:
Look at each positive quality that you wrote down – now describe its opposite (e.g., unfeeling, stingy, dull, etc.):
-
-
-
-
-

Step 3:
Picture a person who embodies these negative qualities vividly in your mind. Roughly speaking, this is your shadow self. Write a description below or draw a picture of your shadow self as you see them here and now:

---

5 *The Mindfulness Solution – Everyday Practices for Everyday Problems* by Ronald D. Siegel.

ACCEPTING AND INTEGRATING YOUR SHADOW SELF

There are many ways to accept your shadow self. Creativity is one of the most therapeutic methods – for example, writing, painting, and dancing with your shadow self. You can also use meditation, breathwork, walks in nature, or any other way that makes you connect with your inner self/higher self.

The most powerful exercise that I use is to write my shadow self a letter using a process called automatic writing.

You begin by writing: 'Dear _____' (your name).

Then continue with:

'Please reveal to me what I am not seeing about my shadow self. What is it trying to guide me to understand? What is it trying to teach me? Please answer me through my pen.'

Take a few breaths and start writing anything that comes through your pen.

Don't look for anything to make sense. Just let streams of thought come through your pen. When the stream of thought ends, read what you have written. You might be surprised.

When working with your shadow self, I recommend practicing automatic writing often. The more you do it, the clearer the messages become.

Use the following page to write a letter to your shadow self.

___

> During this work, the most important thing to remember is that in nature nothing is bad and nothing is good, it just is. We are part of nature so there is nothing bad or good within us, we just are. Our shadow, our light is not bad or good. It just is. We just are.

Dear _____,

_____
_____
_____
_____
_____
_____
_____
_____
_____
_____
_____
_____
_____
_____
_____
_____
_____
_____
_____
_____
_____
_____
_____
_____
_____
_____
_____
_____

With love and appreciation, _____ .

CELEBRATING OSTARA

Akin to Yule, Ostara is one of the festivals on the wheel where ancient Celtic and Nordic traditions have survived throughout human history, although often adapted to suit the time period. Pretty much everything we associate with the holiday of Easter has an ancient root.

The symbol that encapsulates all of the many different themes of Ostara and has been associated with this time of year the most is the egg. In some traditions, the golden orb of the yolk represents the Sun God enfolded by the White Goddess – perfect balance – particularly appropriate to Ostara and the spring equinox, when the world is in balance for just a moment.

And, of course, we humans have been decorating them at this time of year for generations. I like to combine my Ostara egg painting with my goal manifestation process. On the next page you can find out how to do that, if this sounds like it would align with you.

In the *Walking the Wheel of the Year* book (pp.89–95), you will find inspiration for Ostara traditions and crafts that you could incorporate into your own Ostara celebrations.

So, how will you celebrate Ostara?
Here's some space for you to write your ideas:

MANIFESTATION EGG PAINTING AND SEED PLANTING

In order to help you manifest your dreams, you can combine egg painting and planting seeds to assist you in this process. You will need to get your creative hat on. This is a seriously fun and messy process that you can do alone or invite your family and friends to do with you. This is a time-honoured tradition in our house, despite the fact that I am the only person who follows the Wheel of the Year spiritually.

Step 1:

Group your goals into a maximum of three distinct and clear groups.

Try to define them in one sentence/word. For example, if one of your goals is to hold to your responsibility in agreements you make, and another is to take responsibility for your own health, then these two goals could be grouped under 'responsibility'.

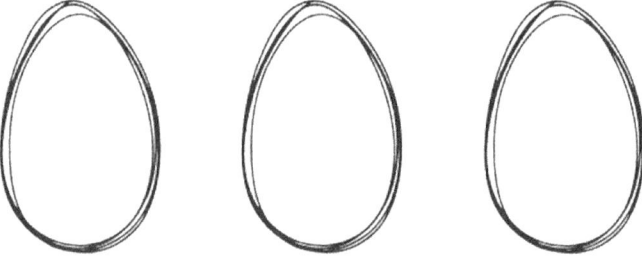

Step 2:

Blow a maximum of three eggs and paint each one to represent your goals.

Remember that your paintings do not have to be masterpieces. Put these eggs in your sacred space to serve as a reminder throughout the year. Each year, I leave my eggs in my sacred space, and then at the next Ostara I grind the old eggshells down and add them to the earth where I plant my new seeds. Each dream fertilizes the next.

SYMBOLISM OF OSTARA

Fertility, abundance, clearing and cleaning, new life, planting seeds, balance, transition, moving from the dark to the light. Integrating the shadow self.

Date of Ostara:

Ostara is celebrated between the 20th, 21st, and 22nd of March. You can celebrate all three days or focus on the actual equinox day.

Symbols of Ostara:

Eggs, seeds, daffodils, lambs, hares, sunwheels.

Colours:

Bright green, yellow, gold, purple (I like to add blue, but it is not traditional).

Foods:

Everything and anything with eggs! Hot cross buns (the perfect sunwheel), honey, leafy greens, dairy foods, nuts, seeds, milk.

Herbs:

Birch, thyme, tarragon, lemon balm, red clover, marjoram, chamomile.

Flowers:

Daffodils, primroses, violets, crocuses, celandine, catkins, pussy willow in profusion (pretty much all early spring flowers), shamrock, dandelion.

Animals:

Birds, lambs, sheep, hare, rabbits, chickens.

Goddesses:

Ostara, Eostre, Frigg, Asase Yaa, Freya, Mother Earth, the Maiden Goddess.

Gods:

The Green Man, Adonis, Cernunnos, Narcissus, Odin, Frey.

CEREMONY PLANNER

What is the purpose/intention of the ceremony?

Where and when will the ceremony be held?

How will I create sacred space (including how the ceremony will start and end)?

What activities will happen during the ceremony (including tools/items needed)?

Words to create sacred space/begin the ceremony[6]:

Words for activities, prayers, gratitude:

Words to end the ceremony:

---

6   It is important to really think through what you want to say in ceremony.

OSTARA JOURNEY

You can find the Ostara Journey in the *Walking the Wheel of the Year* book (pp.97–98). When you have done your journey, as you slowly recover, write down or draw what you can remember from your journey (remember that recovering includes drinking water and eating some good chocolate!).

_____
_____
_____
_____
_____
_____
_____
_____
_____
_____
_____
_____
_____
_____
_____
_____
_____
_____
_____
_____
_____
_____
_____
_____

AS THE WHEEL TURNS...

After Ostara, nature really does get cracking on with the whole growth thing! In Denmark, traditionally the farmers don't begin planting until after Ostara. The birds are nest-building, and buds are bursting open, which means it's time for us to get going too. Hibernation is done – it's now a time for doing!

Here is some inspiration for different activities that you can incorporate into your life until Beltane. As always, these are for inspiration only. Do what makes sense for you and your life.

- Practice the Tree of Life Meditation once a week.
- If possible, take a walk in nature every week to see how quickly the environment changes around you.
- Plant some seeds on a windowsill and in a garden and, as you care for them, remember to nurture yourself and your own growth too.
- Continue to work with your shadow self.
- Begin following your goal action steps.

I wish you a magical and inspiring Ostara!
Blessings,

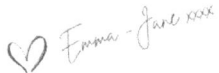

YOUR NOTES

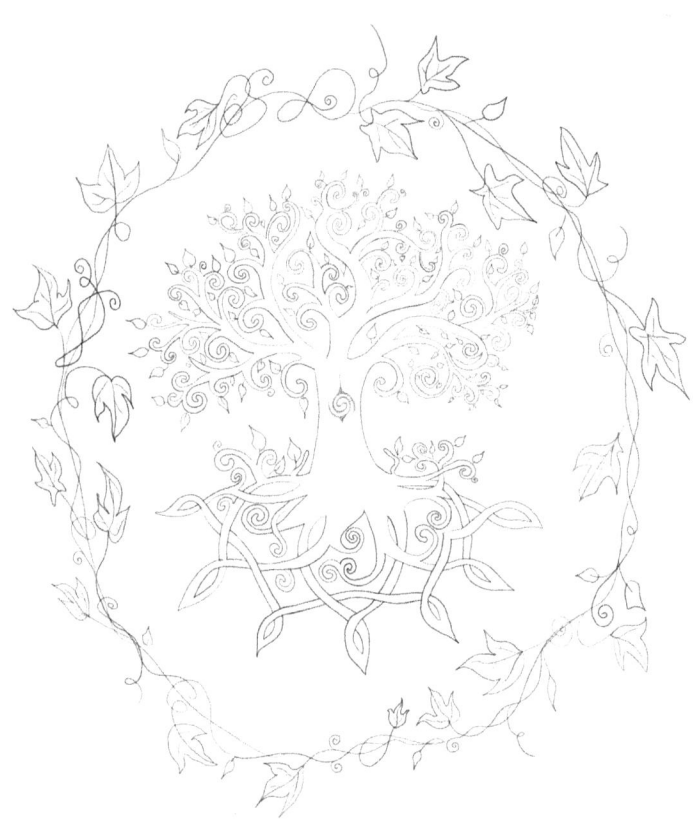

Beltane

31st April/1st May

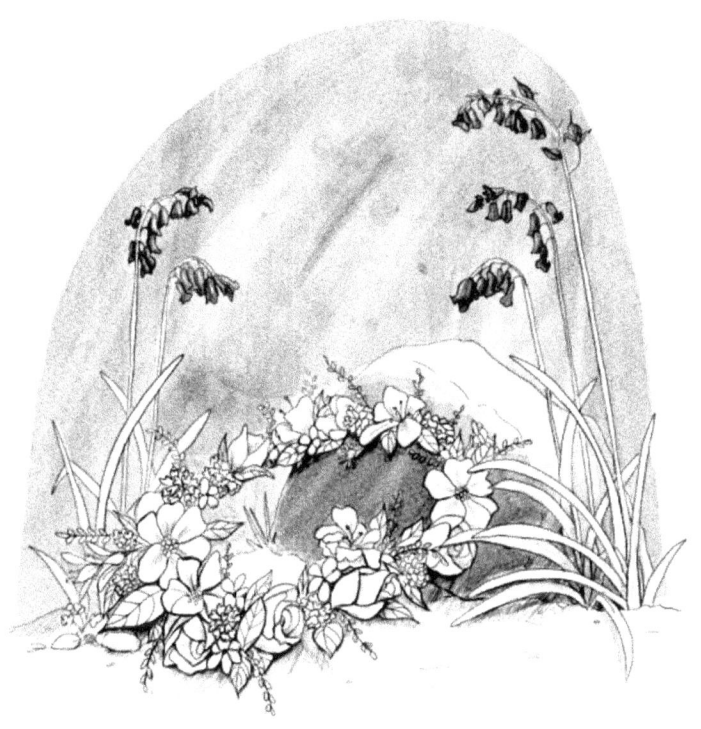

The wheel has turned once more…
The sun warms the land.
Blossoms scent the air,
As you take your love by the hand.

CONNECTING WITH THE SEASON

The wheel has turned, and it is time to reflect and feel into the energy of Beltane. Before you read the chapter on Beltane in the *Walking the Wheel of the Year* book, take a walk alone outside and find a quiet place where you feel comfortable and do the Tree of Life Meditation (p.203).

Now continue your walk. Remember, this is a time to reflect upon nature's journey as the macrocosm, and our journey in life as the microcosm. As you walk, reflect upon the following questions and, when you come home to your sacred space, write down the answers.

How has the world around you changed since Ostara?
_____
_____
_____
_____
_____
_____

How has your life changed since Ostara?
_____
_____
_____
_____
_____
_____

Can you see the connections between nature's changes and your life's changes?

_____
_____
_____
_____
_____
_____

How is this season's energy reflecting where you are in your life right now?

_____
_____
_____
_____
_____
_____
_____
_____
_____
_____
_____

> Now read Beltane: Love and Sensuality – The Dance of Life, in the *Walking the Wheel of the Year* book (pp.99–119).
> You can read just the history and then come back to do the following exercises, or read the entire chapter and then come to this workbook to do the processes.

GROWING WITH THE SEASON

Reflections on working with the shadow self

Where is the best place to begin our self-love journey? By looking at the shadow self. So, let's start from where we left off at Ostara by looking at our relationship with our shadow self. From Ostara to now, you have been journeying to visit and working with your shadow self.

Your understanding of your shadow will have empowered you. It may have opened old wounds or led you to investigate early experiences in your life. If you have peeled back to the deeper layers, then you may have found the root of your insecurities and fears. Now it is time to reflect upon that work and move on.

Journal the answers to the following questions to see how your relationship has changed with your shadow self since Ostara.

How has my relationship with my shadow self developed?

_____
_____
_____
_____
_____
_____

What have I learned about my shadow self?

_____
_____
_____
_____
_____
_____

Do I need/want to continue working with my shadow self for the remainder of this wheel?

_____
_____
_____
_____
_____

Can I accept all that I have learned and understood about my shadow self?

_____
_____
_____
_____
_____

Can I now understand where my shadow self is limiting me / holding me back in my life?

_____
_____
_____
_____
_____

What other thoughts and insights do I have from this work?

_____
_____
_____
_____
_____

WORKING WITH SELF LOVE

Your past inspiring your now

Find photographs of you when you were younger and happy. Choose these pictures from a broad range of your life, such as a baby, a toddler, at age 11, 13, 16, 18, 21, 30, 40, and so on. Also, if you have them, select pictures of significant moments or memories from your life.

Look at the pictures in age order. As you look at each picture, meditate upon it.

- What do you love about this version of you?
- Do you still have or recognise this quality within you today?
- If not, do you want this quality in you today, and how will you bring this into your life now?

Write the qualities upon the back of each photo, or as a list in your workbook.

Now, individually, look at each image again and feel love for the person in the picture.

You can return to these pictures whenever you need to remember the beautiful, unique, perfectly imperfect person you are. Put them in your sacred space.

> Working with self-love is a gradual process. You may not feel the love for yourself all at once. In fact, I would be very surprised if you did. However, if you repeat this process every wheel, then I know that self-love and respect will grow.

Age in picture:
_____

What do I love about this version of me?
_____
_____

Age in picture:
_____

What do I love about this version of me?
_____
_____

Age in picture:
_____

What do I love about this version of me?
_____
_____

Age in picture:
_____

What do I love about this version of me?
_____
_____

Age in picture:
_____

What do I love about this version of me?
_____
_____

Can I see these things in me today and love them?
_____
_____

LOVE LETTER

The voices we hear the most are the ones we believe. The neuroscience of self-talk has taught us that it can form new neural pathways in the brain, essentially becoming something we believe[7]. Evidence has also shown that positive mental and physical outcomes associated with positive and loving thoughts or self-talk enhances self-esteem and confidence[8].

Ergo, negative self-talk or positive self-talk, hateful talk or loving talk – we will believe what we hear the most. On that premise, it is logical that we need to hear words of love from ourselves to ourselves to be able to love ourselves.

One of my favourite ways to do this that I repeat every Beltane is to write a love letter to myself, read it aloud, and then put it in my sacred space. I also keep these love letters, and throughout the years, when I have felt my self-love battery draining, I re-read them.

On the next page, you can write a love letter to yourself.

---

7 BrainFutures 2025 – Neuroplasticity 101. www.brainfutures.org/neuroplasticity-101
8 *The Science of Affirmations: The Brain's Response to Positive Thinking* by Koosis, L.A. www.mentalhealth.com/tools/science-of-affirmations

Dear _____,

_____
_____
_____
_____
_____
_____
_____
_____
_____
_____
_____
_____
_____
_____
_____
_____
_____
_____
_____
_____
_____
_____
_____
_____
_____
_____

I love you, _____.

DAILY SELF-LOVE PRACTICE

Creating a habit of self-love practices is incredibly empowering. From Beltane, I like to do a daily or a weekly self-love worksheet to reinforce these new neural pathways! On the following page, I have included a worksheet for you.

Making time for you

It's all very well and good saying that you must practice self-love. However, we all know that in life's hurly-burly, self-love and self-care can get shoved to low priority on our life's to-do list. I invite you to do this differently, and for the time between Beltane and Litha (20th/21st/22nd June), make self-love the top of your priority list.

What is it that you will do to practice self-love from now until Beltane? List three things below:

-
-
-

Now look at your diary and plan exactly when you are going to take the time to do each of these **things – and keep that time sacred!**

*** If you need inspiration, you can find lots suggestions for self-love practices in the *Walking the Wheel of the Year* book (pp.103–108). ***

Self Love Practice

Describe you kindly

Something that I am proud of

....
....
....
....

Something that Is unique about me

....
....
....
....

A thought i want to think about myself

....
....
....
....
....

Two things to do for myself today

....
....
....
....

Love yourself so fiercely that you show others how it should be done

A feeling I want to practice today

....

Two things I love about myself

....
....
....
....

A compliment to myself

I LOVE ....
(your name)

103

AWAKENING YOUR SENSES

Beltane is the time to awaken your senses. This practice for awakening and exploring the senses is a mindful way to activate and connect with your senses. Make sure to do each step for a period of no less than three minutes.

Sit comfortably and breathe deeply. Keep your eyes open.

Begin to focus on the smallest thing you can see. Experience it. See every detail.

Now begin to focus on the next largest thing you can see. Experience it. See every detail.

Now begin to focus on the largest thing you can see. Experience it. See every detail.

Now begin to focus on everything you can see. Experience it. See every detail.

Close your eyes. Take three deep breaths.

Begin to focus on the smallest noise you can hear. Experience it. Hear every detail.

Begin to focus on the noises you can hear in the room or space you are in. Experience them. Hear every detail.

Begin to focus on the noises you can hear far away from the room or space you are in. Experience them. Hear every detail.

Begin to focus on all of the noises you can hear in the room or space you are in. Experience them. Hear every detail.

Keep your eyes closed. Take three deep breaths.

Focus on your mouth. Taste the feeling inside your mouth.

Keep your eyes closed. Take three deep breaths.

Focus on your body. Feel your connection to the ground. Feel the air on your skin, the warmth.

Now take your hands to your heart and feel your heartbeat. When you are ready, begin to move your body and stretch out.

CELEBRATING BELTANE

Beltane is very much a festival with Celtic roots. Just like Samhain, its opposite on the Wheel, it is celebrated over two days: Beltane Eve on April 30th and May Day on May 1st. The Celts believed that the new day began at sunset[9] – both of these festivals, celebrated from sunset to sun up, represent this ancient Celtic belief. In my experience, it is most potent in feeling the energies of these festivals when celebrating them on the actual day, wherever possible. In Britain, there are many Mayday celebrations, pagan and non-pagan, that are celebrated with the now traditional Maypole dance. If you haven't tried it, I can recommend it. Beltane is truly (for me) a festival where dancing connects you with the land's life-force.

In the *Walking the Wheel of the Year* book (pp.89–95), you will find inspiration for Beltane traditions and crafts that you could incorporate into your own Beltane celebrations.

So, how will you celebrate Beltane?

Here's some space for you to write your ideas:

---

9 Ephemeris.com: History of Astronomy – The Celts. http://ephemeris.com/history/celts.html

SYMBOLISM OF BELTANE:

Love, fertility, self-love, marriage, lust, sexuality, the Fae, divination, handfasting, puberty, maidenhood.

Symbols of Beltane:
Blossom, flowers, maypole, fire, sex, floral crowns, seed, the Fae, sacred bodies of water, wreaths, ribbons, bees, maidens, rose-quartz, hearts.

Colours:
Pink, purple, green, light blue, yellow, white, brown.

Foods:
Honey cakes, sangria, lemonade, strawberries, spring greens, cherries, recipes including milk or dairy products, May bowl (punch).

Herbs:
Mint, lemon balm, willow, birch, hawthorn, woodruff, ivy, mugwort.

Flowers:
Daisies, blossoms, violets, lilacs, roses, snapdragons, jasmine, elderflower.

Animals:
Rabbits, cows, sheep, bees, robins, hawks, frogs, doves, sows.

Goddesses:
Frejya, Maiden Goddesses, Blodewedd, Aphrodite, Arianrhod, Artemis, Astarte, Venus, Diana, Flora, Skadi, Shiela-na-gig, Cybele, Rhiannon.

Gods:
The Green Man, Adonis, Cernunnos, Frey, Pan, Herne the Hunter, Apollo, Bacchus, Bel/Belanos, Faunus, Cupid/Eros, Odin, Orion, Robin Goodfellow, Puck, the Great Horned God.

CEREMONY PLANNER

What is the purpose/intention of the ceremony?

Where and when will the ceremony be held?

How will I create sacred space (including how the ceremony will start and end)?

What activities will happen during the ceremony (including tools/items needed)?

Words to create sacred space/begin the ceremony[10]:

Words for activities, prayers, gratitude:

Words to end the ceremony:

---

10 It is important to really think through what you want to say in ceremony.

BELTANE JOURNEY

You can find the Beltane Journey in the *Walking the Wheel of the Year* book (pp.97–98). When you have done your journey, as you slowly recover, write down or draw what you can remember from your journey.

_____
_____
_____
_____
_____
_____
_____
_____
_____
_____
_____
_____
_____
_____
_____
_____
_____
_____
_____
_____
_____
_____
_____
_____
_____
_____
_____
_____

MANIFESTING YOUR GOALS

You thought I forgot, didn't you! Nope – just after your Beltane celebration is a good time to check in with your goals and your progress so far.

What goals have I been working on since Ostara?

_____
_____
_____
_____
_____
_____

What have I achieved so far?

_____
_____
_____
_____
_____
_____

Which goals and action steps will I work on from now until Litha, the summer solstice?

_____
_____
_____
_____
_____
_____

AS THE WHEEL TURNS...

Beltane energy is infectious and jubilant and not something that can be maintained until Litha, the summer solstice. However, there are many ways to keep yourself connected to the energy of growth and change that happens from now until Litha – and there will be a lot, as nature is building up to its growth crescendo! Here are suggestions of things you can do to stay connected to nature's journey until Litha:

- Practice the Tree of Life Meditation once a week.
- If possible, take a walk in nature every week to see how quickly the environment changes around you.
- Dedicate some time each week to a self-love practice.
- Dance, dance, dance, whenever you can!
- Continue to work with your shadow self.
- Keep following your goal action steps.

I wish you a magical and inspiring Beltane!
Blessings,

Emma-Jane xxx

YOUR NOTES

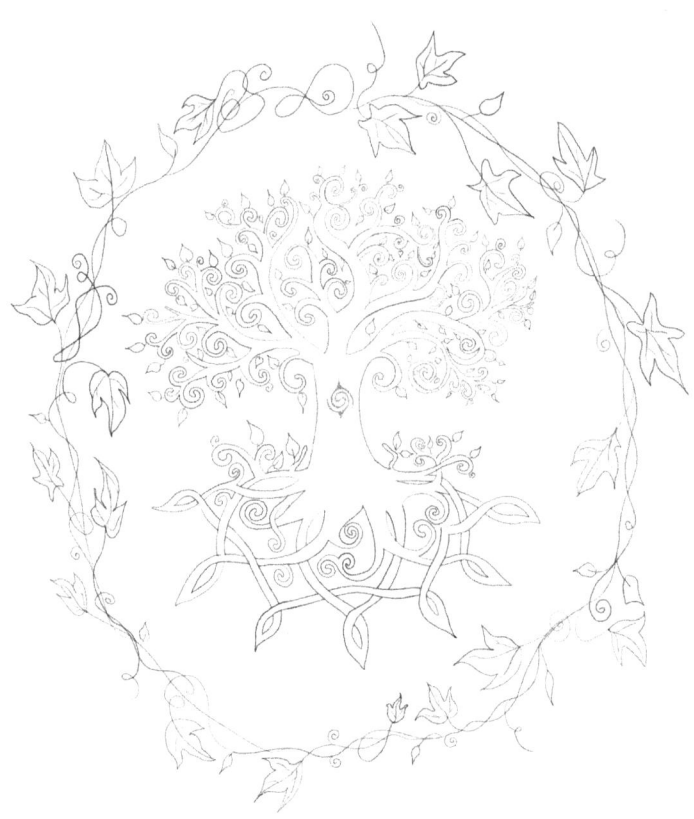

Litha and the Summer Solstice

20th/21st/22nd JUNE

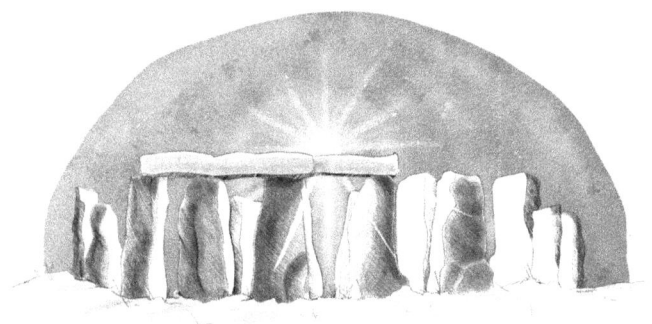

The wheel has turned once more…
The longest day, the shortest night.
We laze in the heat and make merry,
While the summer sun is at its height.

Litha

CONNECTING WITH THE SEASON

The wheel has turned, and it is time to reflect and feel into the energy of Litha, the summer solstice. Before you read the chapter on Litha in the *Walking the Wheel of the Year* book, take a walk alone outside and find a quiet place where you feel comfortable and do the Tree of Life Meditation (p.203).

Now continue your walk. Remember that this is a time to reflect upon nature's journey as the macrocosm, and our journey in life as the microcosm. As you walk, reflect upon the following questions and, when you come home to your sacred space, write down the answers.

How has the world around you changed since Beltane/winter solstice?

_____
_____
_____
_____
_____
_____

How has your life changed since Beltane/winter solstice?

_____
_____
_____
_____
_____
_____

Can you see the connections between nature's changes and your life's changes?

_____

_____

_____

_____

_____

_____

How is this season's energy reflecting where you are in your life right now?

_____

_____

_____

_____

_____

_____

> Now read Litha – The Height of Power, in the *Walking the Wheel of the Year* book (pp.120–122).
>
> You can read just the history and then come back to do the following exercises, or the entire chapter and then come to this workbook to do the processes.

GROWING WITH THE SEASON

Embracing your power
At Litha, the sun is at the pinnacle of its journey, at its full power before the birth of the winter sun. It's time to connect with that energy by reflecting it within yourself and embracing your power.

You are a **powerful self**. Self-power, or empowerment, is the source of energy for your body-mind-psychic centre and intellect, your own personal driving force. When your mind is in harmony with your self-power, your mental stamina becomes stabilized. When we claim our self-power, recognise and own it, then we become empowered in ourselves and in our lives.

And just like self-love, this is not a quick journey. Embracing, acknowledging, even celebrating your power can take a while. Returning to this journey from Litha to Lammas each wheel will make it easier, but if this is your first time, it is ok if it's hard. Stick with it and be gentle with yourself. If you have resistance coming up, then journal everything, because that resistance is your soul's way of trying to alert you to a block to you embracing and recognizing yourself as a powerful being. In the *Walking the Wheel of the Year* book (pp.122–131), there are many, many suggestions of different ways of working with your own power. However, I have included in this journal my go-to tools that I return to each Litha to help me embrace my power.

Why did I create this?
I believe that life, the universe (insert your own name for it here), is often trying to send us teachings to guide us on this earth walk and help us to gain insight into ourselves that allows us to grow. The most important thing about your past is learning from it. Yes, you have made choices, but *everything* in life is an opportunity to learn. When you look back at your life, there will be repeating patterns. These are a huge opportunity for learning.

One tool I was taught was to look at situations from the perspective of 'why did I create this?' – both good and bad situations.

Now, I am not saying that you create everything in your life. Some things we do, some things we don't. However, using this question as a reflection question will help you to understand, learn and grow (particularly the bad situations).

For example, I had a heart attack caused by a disease I didn't know I had. Did I create it? Well, no. But by using this thought process, I realised that I honestly needed a shock to wake me up and get realigned with my values in my life. This book is one of the results from that process.

Try the 5-step process below[11] to see if this tool could be a helpful reflection tool for you. A bit of a warning: I hated using this process when I first used it. It took a while for it to help, so don't worry if it makes you feel uncomfortable. Growing is uncomfortable. Just think how much earth a shoot has to shift to become a plant. That cannot be painless! You got this.

Why did I create this?
Think back to something that has happened in your life. Not a good situation, and not the worst experience you have ever had either – but choose a not-great situation.

1. Write a short sentence explaining what happened:
_____
_____
_____

2. Write why and how this happened to you, whose fault you thought it was:
_____
_____
_____

---

[11] This process is slightly different from the one in the *WTWOTY* book, as I have since altered my own process.

Now we are going to look at your responsibility in this situation by asking yourself:

Why and how did I create this event?

3. Write down in a list the actions you took in this situation:

_____
_____
_____

What was the outcome of these choices/actions?

_____
_____
_____

4. Now write what happened in your life after this event:

_____
_____
_____

Why was this event necessary in your life?

_____
_____
_____

5. What was the teaching you needed to learn from this situation?

_____
_____
_____

YOUR PAST INSPIRING YOUR NOW

Recognising your power can be just as challenging as finding things you can love about yourself, so we are going to repeat the exercise we did at Beltane, but this time we are looking at recognising your power. You can use the same pictures from Beltane or find photos of you when you were younger and happy. Again, make these pictures from a broad range of your life, such as a baby, a toddler, at ages 11, 13, 16, 18, 21, 30, 40, 50, 60, and so on. Also, if you have them, choose pictures of significant moments or memories from your life.

Look at the pictures in age order. As you look at each picture, meditate upon:

- What strengths can you see in this version of you?
- Do you still have or recognise this quality within you today?
- If not, do you want this quality in you today (and how will you bring this into your life now)?

Write the qualities upon the back of each photo or as a list in your workbook.

Now, individually look at each picture again and see the power of the person in the picture.

You can return to these pictures whenever you need to remember the powerful person that you are. Put them in your sacred space.

> *** Like self-love, working with, acknowledging and claiming your personal power is a gradual process. It can also bring up past memories, hurts and fears. If this happens then I recommend using the empty pages at the back of this workbook to free write to the universe and ask what it is trying to teach you from these feelings and what work you need to do to resolve them. If a lot is coming up and you feel overwhelmed, please don't try to do this alone, seek professional support. ***

Age in picture:
_____

What power can I see in this version of me?
_____
_____
_____

Age in picture:
_____

What power can I see in this version of me?
_____
_____
_____

Age in picture:
_____

What power can I see in this version of me?
_____
_____
_____

Age in picture:
_____

What power can I see in this version of me?
_____
_____
_____

Age in picture:

_____

What power can I see in this version of me?

_____

_____

_____

_____

Now write a list of the powers you can see in the past you:

_____

_____

_____

_____

SEARCHING FOR YOUR POWER

One of the best ways to learn about your power is to recognise someone else's power and help them discover it for themselves. If you can find someone you can do this exercise with then take five minutes to ask each other these questions (with a timer set for five minutes[12]):

- What makes you truly happy?
- What are your core personal values?
- What have you done in your life that you are most proud of?
- What is the second thing that you are most proud of?
- What empowers you?
- How would you describe your powerful self?

Now read the other person's answers to them. It is amazing when we hear our own thoughts aloud how differently we perceive them. Reverse the process and listen to your own answers. If you are doing this exercise alone, then make sure you read your answers out loud.

Look at the person you have found yourself to be today. This person is strong. This person needs to be honoured.

What makes you truly happy?

_____
_____
_____
_____
_____
_____

---

12 Using a timer helps us to not over-think and answer with our true unconscious instinct, not our insecurities!

What are your core personal values?

_____
_____
_____
_____

What have you done that you are most proud of?

_____
_____
_____
_____

What is the second thing that you are most proud of?

_____
_____
_____
_____

What empowers you?

_____
_____
_____
_____

How would you describe your powerful self?

_____
_____
_____
_____

MAKING YOUR 'I AM' STATEMENTS

One of the most powerful statements in the world is 'I AM'. In saying 'I am', we are defining ourselves. There is no uncertainty. No room for doubt. 'I am' is a 100% statement of creation. By stating what we are, we are bringing it into reality.

As I wrote at Beltane, the voices we hear the most are the ones we believe. Using 'I am' statements as positive reinforcement will aid in the forming of new neural pathways in the brain and will become what we believe about ourselves.

In looking for your power, you will have seen similar words pop up again and again. Now you are going to use those to create 'I am' statements for the strengths you see in yourself or, if you dare, the strengths other people see in you, for example:

I am brave.
I am strong.
I am kind.
I am caring.
I am creative.
I am a teacher.

On the next page, write out your six 'I am' statements. Make sure you use the full sentence for each one, starting with 'I am'.

Make a list. Pin them by your bathroom mirror and read them out loud every morning from now until Lammas. This will help create those new positive neural pathways.

Over time, hopefully you will begin to notice how much stronger you feel and how rooted and grounded you are in your own identity and power.

I like to combine my 'I am' statements with the craft of making a solstice sunwheel or, as I like creative projects, on the years where I really feel I need my 'I am'-s, I make it a bit of an art project. Have fun with this list.

MY 'I AM' STATEMENTS

BE YOUR OWN PERSONAL TEAM COACH

If you have been working through some of the processes described, then you hopefully will be feeling ultra powerful right now! But, what about next week? Or next month? Motivation is a fickle friend. It can be hard to find this feeling amidst those moments where we feel most powerless. An exercise I found in *The Magic of Thinking Big* by David Schwartz PhD.[13] showed me the perfect way to help the future you. You need to write and read your own team pep talk! When we write and put conscious effort into creating, then it becomes more believable. Re-reading your writing makes your words believable. Yep, we are back to creating those neural pathways again. I did mention this path is about growing, right?!

Create your pep talk

Let me start with the disclaimer that this can feel a bit cringey or faked. Here I will say: trust the process. It is totally ok to toot your own horn and remind yourself how fabulous you are. The universe didn't grow you to be small; it grew you with so much potential and gave you everything you needed to fulfil it.

Begin your pep talk by introducing you to yourself, then starting as many sentences as possible with your name to tell yourself about all the amazing things about you. I write a new pep talk every summer solstice, because I need to hear different things. Read your letter out loud whenever you need to be reminded of your power until next summer solstice, and then make yourself a new one. Write your letter below.

Here is the beginning of one of mine to get you started:

> 'Emma, this is Emma.
> Emma is a wonderful person. She connects with people. Emma inspires people and helps them with their lives. She brings people back to living with nature, to appreciate the world around them. Emma loves the world and is loved in her life. Emma is a wonderful, amazing and beautiful person.'

---

13 *The Magic of Thinking Big* by David Schwartz PhD.

_____ , this is _____ .

_____ is a uniquely powerful being!

CELEBRATING LITHA

Summer solstice is the pinnacle of the sun's journey, and I have always found the shortest night to be one of the craziest nights of the year, energy-wise. I have celebrated Litha at Stonehenge, at Avebury, and alone in a field or on a balcony in Cannes, all over the world in fact; and yet, being outside on the shortest night feels the same everywhere. This truly, in my opinion, is a night to be outside and, if possible, stay awake all night and see the sunset and sunrise.

Of course, droves and droves of people in the UK head towards stone circles for the summer solstice. Which I get is a magical experience. However, I am at heart an eco-witch, and I would ask you not to do this every wheel. As I studied in Avebury, I spent many years volunteering on the land conservation team and saw firsthand the destruction caused simply by so many humans visiting. And I am not just talking about rubbish or erosion. I mean things like flowers left as offerings that have poisoned and killed the sheep that graze in the circle to help maintain the site. Ribbons wrapped around tree branches that damage these ancient beings, so please think before you go, as I know that you, like me, wouldn't want to harm these amazing spaces.

There are many ways to celebrate Litha. In the *Walking the Wheel of the Year* book (pp.131–137), you will find inspiration for Litha traditions and crafts that you could incorporate into your own celebrations.

So, how will you celebrate Litha?

Here's some space for you to write your ideas:

_____
_____
_____
_____
_____

SYMBOLISM OF LITHA

Heat, the sun, celebration of life, summer, strength, courage, power, creativity, inspiration, transition.

Symbols of Litha:
Sun, drumming, sunwheel, bonfires, roses, daisies, all rayed flowers, torches, fairies.

Colours:
Gold, pink, red, yellow, orange.

Foods:
Honey, ale, bread, cheese, edible flowers, fresh fruits and vegetables, lemons, mead & wine, milk, oranges, pumpernickel bread, oatmeal cakes.

Herbs:
Oak, St. John's wort, frankincense, lemon, sandalwood, heliotrope, copal, saffron, laurel, ylang-ylang, chamomile, cinquefoil, elder, fennel, hemp, larkspur, lavender.

Flowers:
Daisies, blossoms, violets, lilacs, roses, snapdragons, jasmine, elderflower, sunflowers.

Animals:
Bees, bears, salamanders, eagles.

Goddesses:
Sol, Sulis Minerva, Litha, Freya, Hestia, pregnant goddesses, Vesta.

Gods:
The Green Man, Balder, the Holly King, Lugh, Apollo, Frey, Thor.

CEREMONY PLANNER

What is the purpose/intention of the ceremony?

Where and when will the ceremony be held?

How will I create sacred space (including how the ceremony will start and end)?

What activities will happen during the ceremony (including tools/items needed)?

Words to create sacred space/begin the ceremony[14]:

Words for activities, prayers, gratitude:

Words to end the ceremony:

---

14 It is important to really think through what you want to say in ceremony.

LITHA JOURNEY

You can find the Litha Journey in the *Walking the Wheel of the Year* book (pp.138–139). When you have done your journey, as you slowly recover, write down or draw what you can remember from your journey (remember that recovering includes drinking water and eating some good chocolate!).

FIND YOUR TOTEM ANIMAL

Spiritually, your personal power can be seen in your totem animal. In the *Walking the Wheel of the Year* book (p.135) is the method I was taught to connect with your totem animal. If you follow this process, then make some notes here about your journey and your totem animal. Once you have put down your initial thoughts, then you can research the symbology of your totem animal (I personally think it is best to form your own ideas and then see how other people interpret it).

_____
_____
_____
_____
_____
_____
_____
_____
_____
_____
_____
_____
_____
_____
_____
_____
_____
_____
_____

MANIFESTING YOUR GOALS

It's that time of the wheel again. Time to check in with your goals and tend to your crops!

What goals have I been working on since Beltane?

_____
_____
_____
_____
_____
_____

What have I achieved so far?

_____
_____
_____
_____
_____
_____

Which goals and action steps will I work on from now until Lammas?

_____
_____
_____
_____
_____
_____

AS THE WHEEL TURNS...

As much as the winter sun is born on the dawn of the summer solstice day, the sun is still beating high in the sky and the powerful growth energy infusing nature is abundant from Litha to Lammas. It is a bit of a strange time because on the one hand the summer gives us a chance to rest before harvest begins, and yet there is still maintenance to be done on our crops or goals. Life doesn't stand still, but at the same time, it does slow down – reminiscent of the time after the winter solstice. So it's a bit of a balancing act. Here are some ways you can stay attuned to nature's energy from now until Lammas:

- Practice the Tree of Life Meditation once a week.
- If possible, take a walk in nature every week to see how quickly the environment changes around you.
- Connect and journey with your totem animal.
- Say your 'I ams' every day.
- Take some rest time outdoors and recharge those batteries.
- Keep following your goal action steps.

I wish you a magical and inspiring Litha!
Blessings,

Emma-Jane xxxx

YOUR NOTES

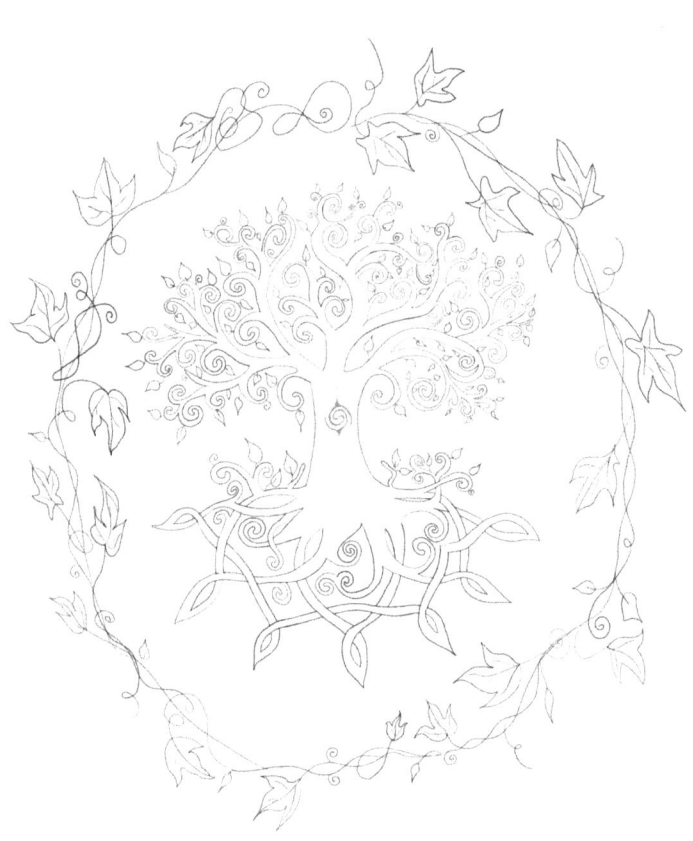

Lammas

1st AUGUST

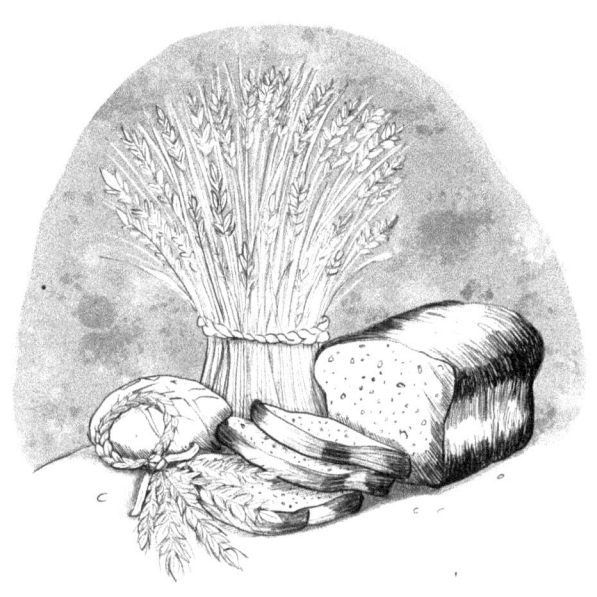

The wheel has turned once more...
The land is golden,
The corn is ripe,
The time to harvest is here...

Lammas

CONNECTING WITH THE SEASON

The wheel has turned, and it is time to reflect and feel into the energy of Lammas, the first harvest. Before you read the chapter on Lammas in the *Walking the Wheel of the Year* book, take a walk alone outside and find a quiet place where you feel comfortable and do the Tree of Life Meditation (p.203).

Now continue your walk. Remember that this is a time to reflect upon nature's journey as the macrocosm, and our journey in life as the microcosm. As you walk, reflect upon the following questions, and when you come home to your sacred space, write down the answers.

How has the world around you changed since Litha?
_____
_____
_____
_____
_____
_____

How has your life changed since Litha?
_____
_____
_____
_____
_____
_____

Can you see the connections between nature's changes and your life's changes?

_____
_____
_____
_____
_____
_____

How is this season's energy reflecting where you are in your life right now?

_____
_____
_____
_____
_____
_____

Now read Chapter 11: Lammas – The First Harvest, Sacrifice and Rebirth, in the *Walking the Wheel of the Year* book (pp.141–160).

You can read just the history and then come back to do the following exercises, or the entire chapter and then come to this workbook to do the processes.

GROWING WITH THE SEASON

Your first harvest

Lammas is the time of the first harvest and for you the midway point in your manifestation journey. Some of the seeds you planted or goals you have been working on will have already bloomed and manifested into your life. This is your first harvest. Sometimes our first harvest will be obvious; sometimes it will surprise us. It may be that your first harvest is something you have not planned but have learnt throughout the wheel. Discovering your first harvest gives you the opportunity to evaluate and celebrate your progress on the journey of manifestation.

Use your Imbolc vision board and your Ostara step-by-step plans to answer the following questions to discover what your first harvest is.

Firstly, cross off steps you have fulfilled on your Ostara plans.

What goals (or action steps) have you completed so far?

_____
_____
_____
_____
_____
_____

Which goals/projects have you not worked upon, not succeeded in, or no longer feel right for you at this time?

_____
_____
_____
_____
_____

Which projects and goals do you no longer wish to work upon?

_____
_____
_____

Which of the goals/projects that you have worked upon have succeeded?

_____
_____
_____

What do you have left to manifest of this year's goals and dreams?

_____
_____
_____

Have you unexpectedly harvested something along the way?

_____
_____
_____

What is your first harvest?

My first harvest is

_____
_____
_____

SACRIFICES

When we work for things we want, then we often have to sacrifice other things. Whether it be time or energy, or physically giving up something. Like our ancestors gave something precious to their gods, we give what is precious to us to manifest.

What sacrifices have you made in order to manifest this wheel's goals?

_____
_____
_____
_____
_____
_____
_____
_____
_____
_____

What is the result of these sacrifices (if apparent)?

_____
_____
_____
_____
_____
_____

Now look at your goals again. It's time to make some more sacrifices. Look at your goals and cross off the ones you don't feel motivated for or that don't feel relevant. Some plants need to have help to remove leaves or deadheads to help them grow further – and this is our deadheading. Of course, keep these ideas in the back of your mind. It may be that the time is not right in your life for these things, and they may be suitable for another point in your life. Or the fact that they are not flowing and are blocked may be a message which is trying to tell you that something else needs to be worked upon first before you can manifest this goal. Additionally, by sacrificing some of your dreams, you are accepting realistically the time you have to work with manifesting your goals at Samhain. Cut things off your list until you have a maximum of three goals left.

Below, write down the three goals that you will continue to work with from now until Samhain:

Goal 1:

_____
_____
_____

Goal 2:

_____
_____
_____

Goal 3:

_____
_____
_____

MAKING A CONSCIOUS SACRIFICE

Making a conscious sacrifice is a way of refocusing your commitment to your goals after the summer. To make a conscious sacrifice to manifest your remaining goals, answer the following questions for each goal:

Goal 1:

What will you have to or are willing to sacrifice to manifest this into a reality in your life?

_____
_____
_____

How will this impact your life?

_____
_____
_____

How and when will you make this sacrifice?

_____
_____
_____

Goal 2:

What will you have to or are willing to sacrifice to manifest this into a reality in your life?

_____
_____
_____

How will this impact your life?

_____

_____

_____

How and when will you make this sacrifice?

_____

_____

_____

Goal 3:

What will you have to or are willing to sacrifice to manifest this into a reality in your life?

_____

_____

_____

How will this impact your life?

_____

_____

_____

How and when will you make this sacrifice?

_____

_____

_____

MANIFESTING YOUR WHEEL'S GOALS

Well, that was a bit heavy, but stick with me, you got this – you have done some really great work! At Lammas, we need to initiate a period of growth. To rededicate and focus on completing the work we started at Imbolc. It is time to commit to action. Let's get manifesting. For each of your remaining goals, answer one simple question:

What do you need to do by Samhain to have manifested this goal (or to get to the level you feel is a success for this wheel)?

_____
_____
_____

When you have clarity in your answers to these questions, then on the next pages make mini-action step plans to achieving your goals (or edit the existing one if it is still applicable and realistic).

> *** A word of caution – don't put yourself under undue pressure here. You have to accept that you have the time you have. So keep your actions realistic and achievable. ***

Goal 1 Action steps:

What do you need to do by Samhain to have manifested this goal (or to get to the level you feel is a success)?

_____
_____
_____
_____
_____

Goal 2 Action steps:

What do you need to do by Samhain to have manifested this goal (or to get to the level you feel is a success)?

_____
_____
_____
_____
_____
_____
_____
_____
_____

Goal 3 Action steps:

What do you need to do by Samhain to have manifested this goal (or to get to the level you feel is a success)?

_____
_____
_____
_____
_____
_____
_____
_____
_____

GETTING SUPPORT

As I said in the *Walking the Wheel of the Year* book, harvesting is a community activity, and it is really difficult to do alone (it's one of the reasons why the autumn half term is called the Tattie Holiday[15], as the school kids would be helping with the harvest). Lammas is a time to reach out to your community for help and support in your manifestation process.

You need to find a person to help you manifest your goals before Samhain. This person is your accountability partner. It should be someone who is motivated in their own life, will be willing to give you some time every week to help you and, IMPORTANTLY, someone who will not let you make excuses. It is really helpful if your accountability partner is also working on their goals, so that you can also become an accountability partner for them.

How to set up an accountability partnership

Give your partner a copy of your goals (and get a copy of theirs, if you are going to be their accountability partner).

Now make an agreement around how your accountability relationship will work. For example, it could be that once a week you are going to be contacted by your partner by SMS, on the telephone, or via social media to check in.

Make sure that your accountability partner knows that their job is to check in and motivate you in fulfilling your goals if you are having challenges. Make them aware that this is not about being an agony aunt or guilt tripping. Of course they can be understanding, but their job is to help you get back on track to the independence of doing the work you need to do to create your goals, projects or dreams. Support to self-help. Ask your partner to make notes of your conversations and send them to you so that you both can keep track of your progress. In the *WTWOTY* book (pp.148–149), you can find some good tips for an accountability partnership.

---

15 A Rite of Passage: Tattie Holidays by Holmes, H. https://blog.scottish agriculturalimplementmakers.co.uk/a-rite-of-passage-tattle-holidays/

TRANSFORMATION

Lammas truly teaches us that nothing stays the same, that everything is in a constant state of transformation. And, as always, as part of nature, we mirror that by constantly transforming whilst on our life journey. As you walk with the wheel each year, you are in the process of transforming into a stronger, conscious and connected you who is attuned to nature's rhythm. You have already transformed from Samhain until now. Let's take a look at that transformation.

What have you learnt about you during this wheel's transformation?

_____
_____
_____

On the next page, draw you or something representing you in the center.

Around the picture write positive statements about you, starting with the phrase:

I was ....

Around the picture write positive statements about you, starting with the phrase:

I am ....

Around the picture write positive statements about you, starting with the phrase:

I can ....

GRATITUDE

All the harvest festivals of the wheel have an element of gratitude. Nature and life truly bless us with their bounty. Part of enjoying your manifesting journey is also celebrating your achievements. Take a moment on this page to write sentences of gratitude for the things you are thankful for in your life right now. Remember to include yourself in this work and to write the full sentence, starting with '**I am grateful for** ....'

CELEBRATING LAMMAS

Lammas is a beautiful celebration of the bounty that the partnership of humans and nature can create together. Two powerful forces – if the relationship is kept balanced. The first harvest is particularly the festival of wheat as it journeys from plant to bread or beer. You may not be a baker (I am not at all). However, the one activity that truly roots you in Lammas energy is making bread (and flatbread counts!). In the *Walking the Wheel of the Year* book (pp.155–156), you can find one recipe for a traditional Lammas loaf. You will also find more inspiration (pp.152–158) for Lammas traditions and crafts that you could incorporate into your own celebrations.

So, how will you celebrate Lammas?

Here's some space for you to write your ideas:

SYMBOLISM OF LAMMAS

The first harvest, gratitude, transformation, community, grain harvest, games, bread.

Date of Lammas:
Lammas is usually celebrated on 1st August.

Symbols of Lammas:
Wheat, grain, John Barleycorn, corn dollies, bread (shaped like a wheatsheaf).

Colours:
Gold, yellow, brown, dark oranges.

Foods:
Bread, porridge, beer, oats, rye bread, honey and honeycomb.

Herbs and flowers:
Meadow sweet, mint, sunflowers, marigolds, poppies, cornflowers, chamomile, yarrow.

Animals:
Bees, bats, calves, hawks, hedgehogs, horses, ravens, crows.

Goddesses:
The Grain Mother, Demeter, Macha, Rhiannon, The Harvest Queen, Frigg, Tailtu.

Gods:
Lugh, John Barleycorn, Llew of the Ready Hand, Odin, Dionysus, Adonis.

CEREMONY PLANNER

What is the purpose/intention of the ceremony?

Where and when will the ceremony be held?

How will I create sacred space (including how the ceremony will start and end)?

What activities will happen during the ceremony (including tools/items needed)?

Words to create sacred space/begin the ceremony[16]:

Words for activities, prayers, gratitude:

Words to end the ceremony:

---

16 It is important to really think through what you want to say in ceremony.

LAMMAS JOURNEY

You can find the Lammas Journey in the *Walking the Wheel of the Year* book (pp.158–159). When you have done your journey, as you slowly recover, write down or draw what you can remember from your journey (remember that recovering includes drinking water and eating some good chocolate!).

REBIRTH

Like transformation, the theme of rebirth is constantly present at Lammas. The seed becomes the wheat. The wheat is cut down and turned into beer. A full rebirthing takes a lot of time, preferably undisturbed privacy, and a lot of experienced support. It is not a process to undertake lightly, and certainly not a process I would recommend pursuing alone. However, to give you an insight into rebirthing, in the *Walking the Wheel of the Year* book (pp.150–151), there is a visualisation of the rebirthing of your own self-image. This visualisation can be repeated whenever you need it.

Make sure you drink a lot of water after this visualisation. It can also be helpful to record how you felt during this visualization.

AS THE WHEEL TURNS...

Lammas is reminiscent of the burst of growth energy from the spring, but in reverse. Life speeds up again after the brief pause of the summer. We have work to do before the winter comes. Here are some ways you can stay attuned to nature's energy from now until Mabon:

- Practice the Tree of Life Meditation once a week.
- If possible, take a walk in nature every week to see how quickly it changes.
- Write a gratitude list and put it in your sacred space.
- Go to a farmers market.
- Collect seeds.
- Keep following your goal action steps.
- Work with your accountability partner.

I wish you a magical and inspiring Lammas!
Blessings,

♡ Emma-Jane xxxx

YOUR NOTES

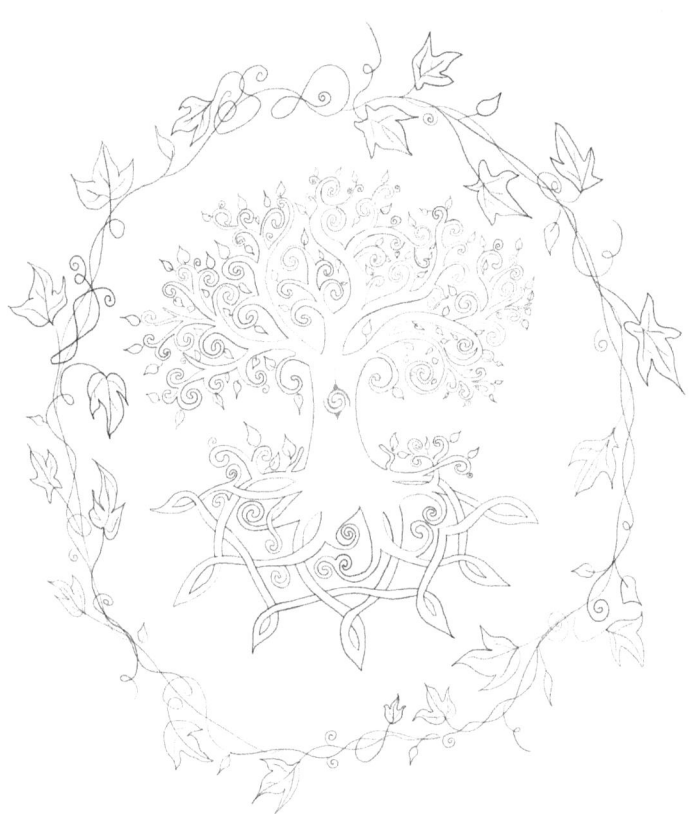

Mabon and the Autumn Equinox

20th/21st/22nd SEPTEMBER

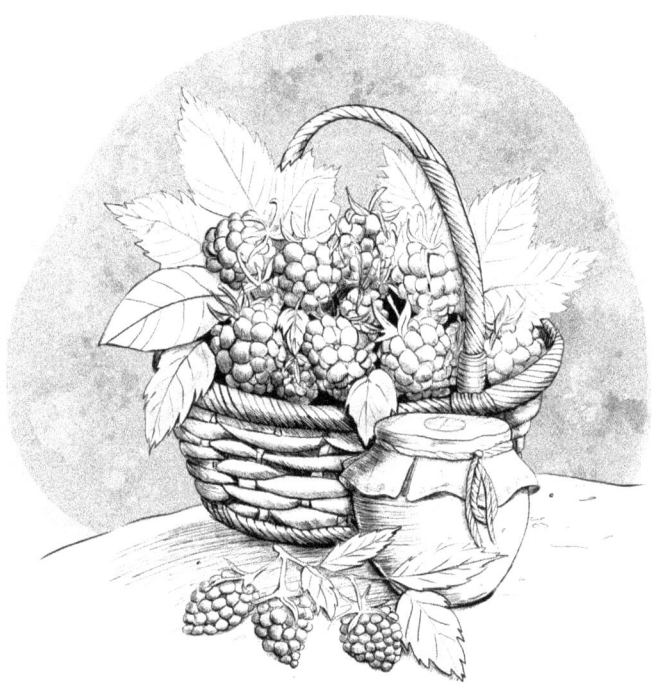

The wheel has turned once more…
We gather the sweetness from the trees.
As the leaves begin to fall,
We can smell winter in the breeze.

Mabon

CONNECTING WITH THE SEASON

The wheel has turned, and it is time to reflect and feel into the energy of Mabon, the second harvest. Before you read the chapter on Mabon in the *Walking the Wheel of the Year* book, take a walk alone outside and find a quiet place where you feel comfortable and do the Tree of Life Meditation (p.203).

Now continue your walk. Remember, this is a time to reflect upon nature's journey as the macrocosm, and our journey in life as the microcosm. As you walk, reflect upon the following questions, and when you come home to your sacred space, write down the answers.

How has the world around you changed since Lammas?
_____
_____
_____
_____
_____

How has your life changed since Lammas?
_____
_____
_____
_____
_____

Can you see the connections between nature's changes and your life's changes?

_____
_____
_____
_____
_____
_____

How is this season's energy reflecting where you are in your life right now?

_____
_____
_____
_____
_____
_____

> Now read Chapter 12: Mabon and the Autumn Equinox – Entering the Dark, in the *Walking the Wheel of the Year* book (pp.161–163).
> You can read just the history and then come back to do the following exercises, or the entire chapter and then come to this workbook to do the processes.

THE SECOND HARVEST

Mabon is the second harvest of the wheel and truly a time of gratitude and celebrating the abundance in our lives. By taking time to reflect upon them, you gain deeper appreciation for yourself and this amazing universe that we live in.

Reflecting on your harvest

Use the following questions to help you reflect on your harvest and your goal manifestation process of the wheel.

What new things have happened in the last year that you are happy with and want to keep in your life (this can include people or other changes)?

_____
_____
_____
_____
_____
_____

What is currently present in your life that you wish would work better or flow more abundantly?

_____
_____
_____
_____
_____
_____

What have you been working on that has not yet manifested (shown up) for you?

_____
_____
_____
_____
_____
_____

What is it that has inspired and supported you throughout this wheel?

_____
_____
_____
_____
_____
_____

What have you discovered about yourself?

_____
_____
_____
_____
_____
_____

PRIDE

During this wheel, you have come to know yourself better, succeeded in following your dreams and made steps to grow as a person and reconnect with the natural world.

You have dedicated yourself to living consciously and mindfully and to being responsible for your path in life. This is a beautiful thing. You may have even surprised yourself along the way. Actually, I hope you have!

It's time for you to acknowledge this journey. A great way to do this is to celebrate everything that you are proud of yourself for on this wheel by acknowledging it.

Write out sentences starting with the phrase:

I am proud of myself for......................

You can do this either on the following blank page, or you can, if you like, make a separate list and put it in your sacred space. Remember to start each point on the list with the words above.

> *** Be proud of your struggles as well as your triumphs. After all, these make up the journey – and the journey is the important part, not the destination.
> And be proud of the small things. We don't have to just celebrate big achievements. Getting out of bed and showing up when we are struggling is just as much something to be proud of as the greatest professional accolade. ***

PRESERVING THE SWEETNESS WITH GRATITUDE AND CELEBRATION

Gratitude and celebration for your bounty are at the heart of the equinox. Gratitude can also be a way of celebrating your achievements. The equinox is about harvesting the sweet things in life and taking stock of what you have harvested so that you know what you have to help you through the winter. So, you are going to make a harvest list celebrating what you are grateful for and what you have accomplished.

Firstly, brainstorm the answers to the following questions:

- What are you grateful for here and now?
- What is the harvest of this wheel?
- What makes your life feel abundant?
- What are your happiest memories of this wheel?

Now fill the next blank page with a list of all the things that you are grateful for and the happy memories you would like to keep as the wheel turns, as well as the things that you are proud of yourself for. I call this a 'Ta-Dah! list' – as in, 'Ta-Dah! Look at what I did!' Then take a look at your harvest, even read it out loud. Look at everything you did and recognise how amazing you truly are.

What are you grateful for here and now?

_____
_____
_____
_____
_____

What have you harvested throughout this wheel?

What makes your life feel abundant?

What are your happiest memories of this wheel?

MY TA-DAH! LIST

REWARD YOUR SUCCESSES

Whilst working with your accountability partners, hopefully they have been reminding you to reward yourself for all of your successes this year. But, you also need to give yourself permission to celebrate without anyone else reminding you to do it. It's time to decide how you are going to reward yourself for the work that you have done on this wheel.

Here and now, decide what you will reward yourself with at Samhain to celebrate your work.

I am going to

- _____

- _____

- _____

as a reward to myself for my work, dedication and growth during this wheel of the year.

*** Make sure you do this before Samhain. No matter how busy your life is, taking time to celebrate you and your life is one of the most important things in life and the most often and easily forgotten. ***

BEING SWEET TO OUR BODIES – PRESERVING OUR STRENGTH

At the autumn equinox, we need to preserve strength and sweetness throughout the darker times. We have a whole winter to get through. And although these days it is easier than ever before, biologically we still need our strength to do it. One of the ways of helping ourselves is to preserve our mental and physical health.

Modern life doesn't support these needs. If you look at the media and advertising focus today, they remind us to get ready for summer. However, it is really winter when we need physical and mental health. The coming winter will also give us much-needed downtime. Downtime is part of the growing period. We need to re-energize to be able to grow in spring.

In the *WTWOTY* book (pp.165–167), you can find lots of inspiration for preserving your strength throughout the winter. You don't have to begin this now, but preparation for the winter is part of the second harvest, so it's good to have your ideas ready.

Below, write some ideas you have to preserve your strength for the winter and what preparation might be needed:

_____
_____
_____
_____
_____
_____
_____
_____
_____

LETTING GO OF OUR SEEDS

Equinox is also the time of seeds being released as the wind scatters them across the earth to grow in the next wheel. Looking at our harvest at the equinox can be both a joyful and sad process. We have the chance to be proud of our accomplishments. However, we are also faced with the regrets and acceptance of unfinished projects or goals unmet. Acceptance makes us stronger. We begin to realise that it is ok to be imperfect. In fact, it's natural.

Here at the equinox, that which we really cannot act upon or manifest before Samhain has to be left behind, ready to be picked up at another time. It is time to ask yourself: what will you let go of before Samhain? What will be the seeds you release?

Choose all but one of your goals to let go. Now fill in the commitment below:

I choose to let go of my dream/goals of

_____

_____

from now until Imbolc. I trust the universe to guide me to manifest this in my life if it is necessary for me. By letting go of

_____

_____

I give space and energy to the process of manifesting

_____

_____

I trust the universe to guide me to manifest this in my life.

BALANCE

The equinoxes are a time of balance, a moment of equal day and night, where the world is in perfect unity. Day and night reflect each other, and at this time we have the biological need to balance within ourselves, reflecting the balance with the world around us. As I said at Ostara, the time before the solar festivals can often feel emotionally wobbly. So, balancing right now is really important to help you feel grounded. There are many practical ways to rebalance yourself. It is important to balance yourself both internally and externally.

One of the best ways to balance yourself internally is to rebalance your chakras. When working with the chakras, each one has a different colour and a different interpretation. Some say that you cannot balance the chakras without visualising the colours. However, I was taught to work with the chakras using first a white light to represent each one. It worked for me, especially as trying to remember the colour sequence took energy from the balancing that I was trying to achieve. Now I use both, whatever fits my mood for that day. On the next page, I have included my version of a chakra rebalancing for you to try. This may not resonate with you, and that is completely fine. The internet has a multitude of different balancing and chakra meditations to try. I also sometimes prefer to use an elemental balancing meditation.

CHAKRA BALANCING MEDITATION

Sit in a comfortable position, preferably connecting with the floor.

Begin to breathe slowly and with purpose, in through your nose and out through your mouth.

Now, from the base of your spine, in a deosil direction (with the movement of the sun), visualise a root connecting and growing downwards to the earth.

Once connected and grounded within the earth, feel energy rising up your roots and into your first base chakra.

Allow the light to slowly start to spiral and spin within your chakra. The light cleans away any dark cobwebs within your chakra. As it spins faster and faster, feel cleansed and energised here in your base chakra.

Repeat this process for all of your chakras, remembering not to stop the previous chakras spinning.

Once you reach your crown chakra, you are in perfect balance. Now, you can choose to allow the energy to burst out of your crown chakra and return like golden rain to the earth, or to begin closing your chakras.

To close your chakras, you begin with slowing down the spinning, sending the energy in a widdershins direction (the opposite movement to the sun). When the spinning has stopped, find a way to imagine your chakra closing. Some people use the image of a flower closing for the night.

Once closed, repeat the process with all of the other chakras until you reach your base chakra.

Once this is closed, return the energy to the earth and slowly visualise the root you planted returning to you from the earth.

WORKING WITH OUR LIGHT SELF

As much as the equinoxes are about balance, they are also about transition from dark to light at the spring equinox and from light to dark here at the autumn equinox.

Working with our light self is equally as important as working with our shadow self, and, sometimes, a little harder. It can be challenging to see our light, but believe me, it is seen by others, and that is the starting point of embracing our inner light.

There are many different ways you can work with accepting and honouring your inner light. In the *Walking the Wheel of the Year* book (pp.169–171), there is inspiration for nurturing your light self. However, my favourite way, other than journeying to meet my light self, is to do the following meditation.

Access my inner light meditation

Here is a simple meditation practice that you can do to access your inner light:

Find a quiet space where you know you won't be disturbed.

Sit comfortably with a nice tall spine, eyes closed and your hands resting in your lap, palms open.

Begin by taking several long, deep, full breaths (down into your belly).

Visualise a beautiful light at your heart space and begin to visualise that light within your heart (keeping your focus and attention on this light).

When the mind wanders, simply return it to this beautiful light in your heart.

Silently repeat the mantra 'my inner light shines' as you focus on the light at your heart space.

Stay here in this space of your heart for a few minutes, repeating the mantra silently and focusing on the light in and around you.

When you are ready to move out of meditation, sit quietly, taking a few moments breathing with ease before moving out into the rest of your day.

CELEBRATING MABON

Mabon is such a beautiful time in the wheel. The last hurrah of life and growth and, at the same time, the beginning of winter's death. It truly is a reminder of the full circle journey we take through the seasons of our lives throughout each and every wheel. And this is a busy time of preparation for the winter too. There are so many ways to celebrate this time. In the *Walking the Wheel of the Year* book (pp.155–156), you can find one recipe for a traditional Lammas loaf. And you will also find more inspiration for Mabon traditions and crafts that you could incorporate into your own celebrations (pp.171–176).

So, how will you celebrate Mabon?

Here's some space for you to write your ideas:

_____
_____
_____
_____
_____
_____
_____
_____
_____
_____

SYMBOLISM OF MABON

Fruit harvest, berry harvest, the second harvest, gratitude, abundance, balance.

Symbols of Mabon:
Berries, the cornucopia, horn of plenty, apples, nuts, seer, sunwheel, preserves.

Colours:
Dark brown, burnt orange, deep green, dark red, golden yellow, earth tones.

Foods:
Berries, pumpkins, apples, corn, zucchini, squash, acorns/nuts, root veggies.

Herbs:
Bay laurel, sage, yarrow, cinnamon, sandalwood.

Flowers:
Rosehips, sunflowers.

Animals:
Stags, owls, blackbirds, squirrels.

Goddesses:
Earth Mother Goddess, Modron, Gaia, Morgan, Epona, Persephone, Demeter, Pomona.

Gods:
Frey, Thoth, Thor, Hermes, Herne the Hunter, the Horned God, the Green Man.

CEREMONY PLANNER

What is the purpose/intention of the ceremony?

Where and when will the ceremony be held?

How will I create sacred space (including how the ceremony will start and end)?

What activities will happen during the ceremony (including tools/items needed)?

Words to create sacred space/begin the ceremony[17]:

Words for activities, prayers, gratitude:

Words to end the ceremony:

---

17 It is important to really think through what you want to say in ceremony.

MABON JOURNEY

You can find the Mabon Journey in the *Walking the Wheel of the Year* book (pp.177–178). When you have done your journey, as you slowly recover, write down or draw what you can remember from your journey (remember that recovering includes drinking water and eating some good chocolate!).

_____
_____
_____
_____
_____
_____
_____
_____
_____
_____
_____
_____
_____
_____
_____
_____
_____
_____
_____
_____
_____
_____
_____
_____
_____

MANIFESTING YOUR GOALS

One goal left to manifest before Samhain. It is a good idea to evaluate your progress with your accountability partner. The time between Mabon and Samhain is shorter than we think. So, you need to really hone in on what are the most important actions that you are going to take during this time.

What goals have I chosen to manifest by Samhain?
_____
_____
_____

What have I done so far?
_____
_____
_____

What action steps do I need to take from now until Samhain?
_____
_____
_____

AS THE WHEEL TURNS...

Although there is more work to do before Samhain, make sure you take the time to pause here at Mabon and truly enjoy the sweetness of your life. Here are some ways you can keep connected to that energy from now until Samhain.

- Practice the Tree of Life Meditation once a week.
- If possible, take a walk in nature every week to see how quickly it changes.
- Make a leaf mandala.
- Cook or preserve with autumn berries or fruits.
- Collect seeds.
- Connect with your light self.
- Prepare anything that you need to strengthen your physical and mental health during winter.
- Keep following your action steps.
- Work with your accountability partner.

I wish you a magical and inspiring Mabon!
Blessings,

Emma-Jane xxxx

YOUR NOTES

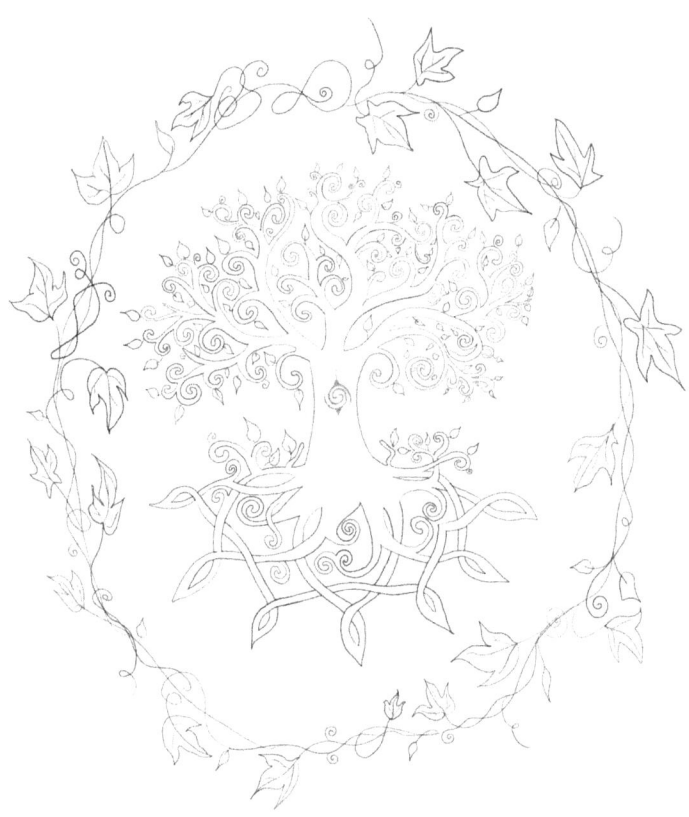

Samhain

31st OCTOBER

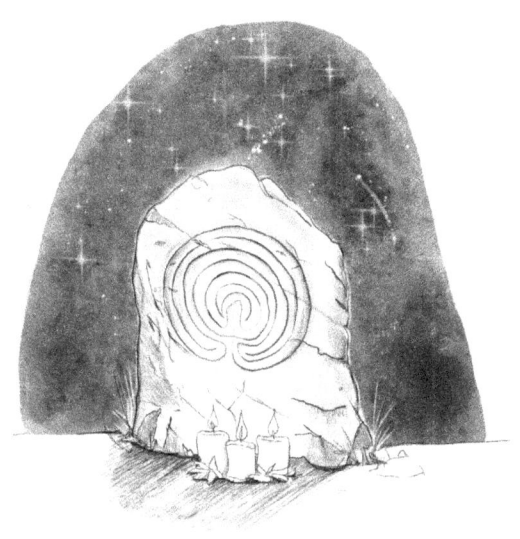

The wheel has turned full circle,
The veils grow thinner.
We celebrate with our ancestors,
And prepare to survive the coming winter…

Samhain

HONOURING THE CYCLE OF DEATH AND REBIRTH

Connecting with the season

Before you read the chapter on Samhain in the *Walking the Wheel of the Year* book, take a walk alone outside and find a quiet place where you feel comfortable and do the Tree of Life Meditation (p.203).

Now continue your walk. As we walk at each festival, this is a time to reflect upon nature's journey as the macrocosm, and our journey in life as the microcosm. It is a moment to bring yourself into flow with the season. As you walk, reflect upon the following questions, and when you come home to your sacred space, write down the answers to the following questions.

> *** Remember to look for the signs of <u>this</u> Samhain, not the signs that you would expect to be looking for. We tend to have preconceived ideas of what each season 'should' look like in nature and in our lives. There is no 'should', and with climate change, the seasons are starting to look very different each year. To attune to nature, we have to look beyond our preconceptions and see what is happening here and now. ***

How has the world around you changed in the last 12 months?
_____
_____
_____

How has your life changed in the last 12 months?

_____

_____

_____

Can you see a connection between your life's journey and nature's journey this wheel?

_____

_____

_____

> Now read Chapter 13: Samhain – The Ending and the Beginning, in the *Walking the Wheel of the Year* book (pp.180–184).
>
> Remember that the exercises in this chapter of your workbook are to be combined with the Samhain exercises at the beginning of the book. If you need a refresher on the historical interpretation of Samhain, then you can read Chapter 5: Samhain – Honouring the Cycle of Death and Rebirth, in the *Walking the Wheel of the Year* book (pp.27–41).

GROWING WITH THE SEASON

The story of your wheel

As you have walked this wheel, you have taken a journey, connected with the land's energy, and made observations about yourself and that of nature. You now have a deeper understanding of the Celtic and Nordic beliefs surrounding the festivals that mark the turning of the seasons, and you have learnt tools and techniques to tune in and connect with each of these. You have also taken a spiritual journey each time within the lower, middle, and upper worlds of your spirit world tree. And in between each festival, you have worked with the energy of the seasons, with your own personal growth and goals. The different activities are parts of your story of this past wheel, recorded in this book or a journal.

Samhain is a good point to look back and acknowledge the journey you have taken before you spiral into the new wheel. To remember this journey, it helps to record it so that you can continue to look back to enrich your understanding, live a conscious life and enjoy your journey. By doing this, you will get an understanding of your own growth rhythm by noticing commonly occurring themes at the same point each wheel. Similarly, you will begin to notice shifts and changes as your own life ebbs and flows through the different stages of this earthwalk journey.

Like the seasons, we all have our own spiral of growth, our own rhythm throughout the seasons that is unique to us. This can take a few wheels to understand as, like nature, we do not follow a specific pattern in our growth each year. Repeating the following exercise each year or every three years will allow you to create a guideline similar to the Wheel of the Year but for yourself.

You are going to create the story of your wheel to help you start to identify your spiral of growth throughout the seasons. Don't get into your head about this. You are not trying to create an epic saga. Your aim is to create something that helps you remember how you ebb, flow and grow throughout the seasons. You can do this with both words and images.

CREATING YOUR STORY

Step 1:
Draw the wheel divided into eight parts and write the names of the festivals by each section. Alternatively, you can use the template on the next page.

Step 2:
Brainstorm what you remember from this wheel's journey for each of the festivals. Include anything that you remember, including life events, and add keywords and symbols that represent these memories. So, if you were feeling very sad at Imbolc, you could use a sad face emoji.

Step 3:
Now look through this workbook or your journal, at your notes from this wheel, and add to your brainstorm anything you remember as being significant for you. It could be your observations, your journeys, your realisations, the goals you have achieved, the craftings we made, or memories from the workshops.

Step 4:
From these notes, create your story for this wheel. Imagine yourself telling the story to someone (it helps to keep it short).

*** The first time you do this, it may seem a little strange, but as you do this process year after year, the patterns will emerge. ***

MY WHEEL

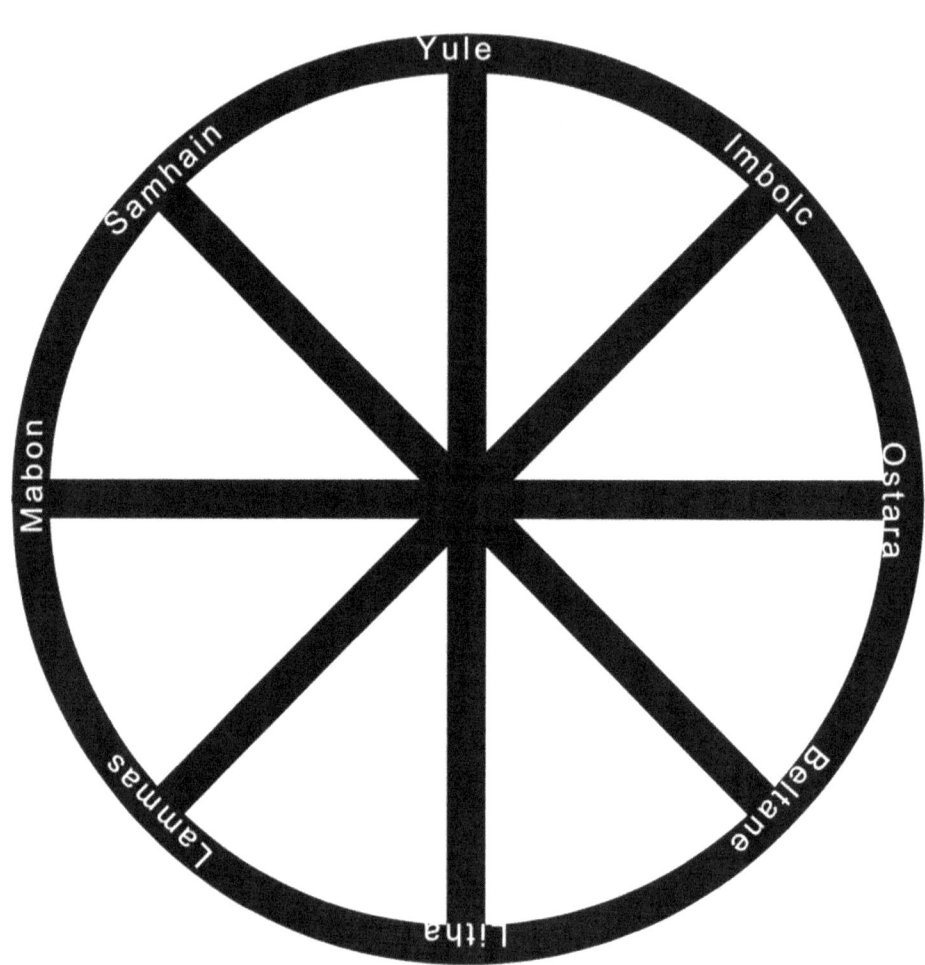

STORY OF MY WHEEL

YOUR MANIFESTATIONS

After Samhain, you may choose to down tools and stop working on your goals for the winter, just as our ancestors did because the growing season ended. Alternatively, you may continue your manifestation journey. If you do, then please be mindful that winter is the time of rest and rejuvenation. Everything slows down, so allow yourself that slow time and rest where you can.

Just as at Mabon, I think it is relevant to be extremely proud of yourself at Samhain. After all, you have been working and growing throughout the whole wheel. Choose the things that you are most proud of, and fill in the blanks of the following sentence below:

I am most proud of myself for………………………………….. **in this, my**………………………… **(year date) journey.**

SUSTENANCE FOR THE DARK TIMES

At Samhain, we celebrate the last of the three harvest festivals. Food was preserved by our ancestors to sustain their families. To complete this wheel's manifestation journey, you need to look at what will give you substance throughout the winter.

Look back at your vision board. One of your goals will be the one that you repeatedly turned to throughout the wheel. It is the goal you have the most passion for, the one that brings the most joy and happiness into your life. It may be that this goal is complete or incomplete. However, it is the one that resonates with you the most. And, most importantly, it is the goal that gives you the most energy. As we turn to the winter, this work will be your sustenance. It will be this that keeps the hearth fire burning in your soul in the dark of winter.

Record your winter sustenance and create a list of things you will do to make it important for you throughout the winter.

My winter sustenance will be:

-
-
-

What will I do to connect with this?

-
-
-

GROWING WITH THE SEASON

Now you can choose which of the Samhain activities from the first Samhain chapter that you wish to do. You can choose to work with letting go, honouring your ancestors as well as the work you have done already. However, remember that you can pick and choose at each festival to do the activities that feel most relevant for you. If you feel that you would like to just do a ceremony or a journey and not the other activities, then that is completely fine.

CELEBRATING SAMHAIN

Of course, every festival needs a celebration. In the *Walking the Wheel of the Year* book (pp.32–36), you will find inspiration for Samhain traditions and crafts that you could incorporate into your own Samhain celebrations.

So, how will you celebrate Samhain?

Here's some space for you to write your ideas:

CEREMONY PLANNER

What is the purpose/intention of the ceremony?

Where and when will the ceremony be held?

How will I create sacred space (including how the ceremony will start and end)?

What activities will happen during the ceremony (including tools/items needed)?

Words to create sacred space/begin the ceremony[18]:

Words for activities, prayers, gratitude:

Words to end the ceremony

---

18 It is important to really think through what you want to say in ceremony.

SAMHAIN JOURNEY

You can find the Samhain Journey in the *Walking the Wheel of the Year* book (p.37). When you have done your journey, as you slowly recover, write down or draw what you can remember from your journey (remember that recovering includes drinking water and eating some good chocolate!).

JOURNEYING IN THE FUTURE

Throughout this wheel, we have journeyed through the World Tree. In the dark half of the year, we journeyed in the cave. In the light half of the year, we journeyed in our grove. And once, at summer solstice, we travelled in our highest plane. From here on, it is up to you how you journey and decide what the purpose is for your journeys. I like to use the following themes in my seasonal journeys, but sometimes my totems have another idea about what we are going to do, so I let them lead me. They generally know best.

Samhain: In my cave I invite my ancestors.

Yule: In my cave I reconnect with my inner child.

Imbolc: In my grove I search for inspiration.

Ostara: From my grove I take a journey to visit my shadow self.

Beltane: In my grove I celebrate Beltane and allow my spirit guides to reveal whatever it is that I need to know.

Litha: In my upper world I connect with the source of my power. Additionally, I sometimes take a separate journey to meet my spirit animal.

Lammas: In my grove I search for inspiration.

Mabon: From my grove I take a journey to visit my light self.

When journeying alone, it is important to remember the guidelines in the journeying and visualisation chapter of the *Walking the Wheel of the Year* book. And don't forget to have some good chocolate on hand for grounding!

AS THE WHEEL TURNS...

As I said in the previous Samhain chapter – of all the festivals, Samhain is really the festival of reconnecting with your roots. Rooting is truly about learning about the foundations of who you are and honouring them.

Here is some inspiration for different rooting activities that you can incorporate into your life until Yule. As always, these are for inspiration only. Some activities go deeper, some don't. Do what makes sense for you and your life.

- Practice the Tree of Life Meditation once a week.
- Visit family and friends.
- Look through old photographs and reflect upon where you came from.
- Free-write in a journal about your roots and your reflections.
- Research your family history.
- Visit ancient sites or woodlands.
- Revisit activities you used to enjoy to see what they bring to you.
- Celebrate your manifestations from this wheel.
- Connect with your sustenance.

I wish you a magical and merry Samhain!
Blessings,

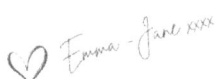

YOUR NOTES

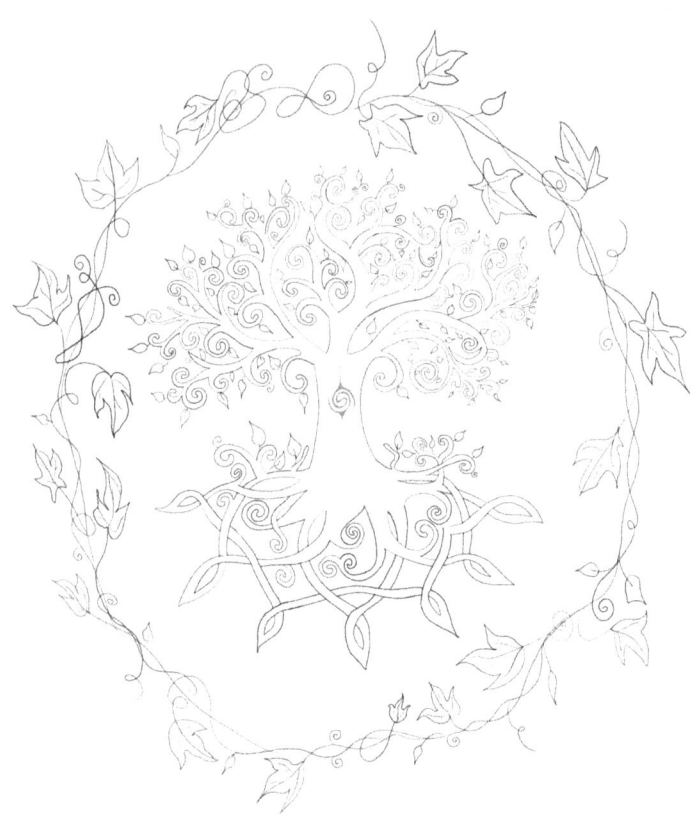

WALKING THE WHEEL OF THE YEAR FROM NOW ON

It has been an honour and a pleasure to share this wheel with you. If you would like more support and community to celebrate the festivals with, then you are also welcome to join my online community, the 'Wheel of the Year – Following the Rhythm of Nature' Facebook group. There you will find a like-minded group of people who have the same respect for nature and understanding of its cycle as you. And of course, you can come to Re:Root Wheel of the Year workshops and gatherings in Denmark and the UK. In the Wheel of the Year Facebook group, you will find information about these events.

Additionally to the book and workbook, if you would like to walk the wheel with me, then you are very welcome to join my Walking the Wheel of the Year online course available at:

www.rerootyourlifecourses.podia.com

Please remember though, the most important thing is that you draw inspiration from my books and courses to find your own way to re-root with nature – because your way is the right way for you. As I said in the *Walking the Wheel of the Year* book:

> 'When you need it, nature is there to guide you – whether in the roots of the trees, the crevices in the stone, the foam on the wave, or the scent in the wind. You are a part of nature. Nature is your wisest teacher, and you are nature's guardian. As she supports us, so we take care of her. So we can grow together…'

My greatest wish for you is that as you re-root with nature, you re-root within yourself, which in time will allow you to re-route your life and make the most of that journey.

Because I truly believe that the most important thing in life is to enjoy the journey!

ADDITIONAL RESOURCES

- Tree of Life Meditation.
- Recommended Reading.
- Tree of Life Mindful Colouring.

*** If you would like a free printable version of the ceremony planner or the self love worksheet these can be found at:

https://rerootyourlifecourses.podia.com/walking-the-wheel-of-the-year-companion-journal-free-printables

Please note, you are welcome to use these worksheets for your own private use but not for commercial purposes. ***

The Tree of Life – the gateway to connection

Stand with closed eyes and begin to breathe slowly and deeply.

From your feet, imagine a root growing deep down within the earth. Feel the wet, moist soil; smell the musky earth. Feel your roots grow and spread until you are fully anchored in the earth.

As your roots reach closer to the centre of the earth, you can see a bright ball of energy at the heart of the planet. Vibrant life energy. As your roots connect to this energy, begin to draw life energy up the roots. Feel the energy nourishing your roots. See them glowing vibrantly.

Draw this energy up towards your feet until you can feel the roots from your feet connected to the earth and the vibrant energy pulsating beneath.

With your next breath, begin to draw the energy upwards. Feel the earth's energy filling your body through your legs. And as the energy connects with your feet and your legs, see them beginning to transform into the trunk of a tree.

Feel the energy rise to your hips, to your stomach. Allow yourself to strengthen your trunk and become stronger, wider. Deeply rooted in the earth and connected to the centre.

Allow the earth energy to rise to your heart. Allow it to spiral slowly, refreshing you. Take a moment here to feel your strength, your connection.

With your next breath, send the energy from your heart through your arms and head. From here, feel your branches begin to form, reaching for the sunlight above. Feel the sap rising up into your branches, revitalising and refreshing you. Allow your branches to spread as wide as your roots, connecting with the sky energy and drawing it in to your heart.

At your heart centre, the earth and the sky energy spiral together. You are balanced between earth and sky. Rooted in the earth. Reaching for the sky. Slowly, leaves begin to grow from the branches, unfurling, warming in the light.

Feel the warmth of the sun as you stand there as a strong tree in the woods. Stand for a while, fully feeling the balance of your branches and your roots. As you stand there rooted in the earth, rain begins to fall, running down your branches, bringing new life to your form.

The rain seeps into the earth, feeding your roots, giving a second surge of energy up into your roots, into your trunk and to your branches.

Now feel the wind gently whistling in your branches. The cold hits the air. Your leaves begin to change colour – bronze, gold, brown and red. With a breath, let them fall to the earth and allow them to rot.

Stand in your winter tree form. Feel the sap retreating from your branches. Release your connection with the sky and draw your arms back in towards your heart. When you reach your heart, you stand once more as a human in your upper body and a trunk below. You can still feel within yourself the balance of the earth and sky energy within your heart.

With your next breath, send the energy down your body to your stomach, your hips, your legs, your ankles until you are standing once more in your human form, yet still deeply connected to the earth by your roots.

As you stand here, you can still feel the balance that you had as a tree between earth and sky. Take a moment to feel that connection.

With your next breath, release your connection to the earth's centre. Leaving with gratitude withdraw your roots back up to your feet until you are once again standing on the earth, no longer rooted, yet still feeling that deep connection, still feeling the balance you felt between the earth and sky, remembering the connection you felt as a tree.

Once you are entirely in your body, slowly begin to open your eyes and breathe normally. If you are outside, look at nature around you. If indoors, then look out of the window. If possible, take a walk and look for the signs of the seasons and meditate upon your journey as part of nature.

TREE OF LIFE MINDFUL COLOURING

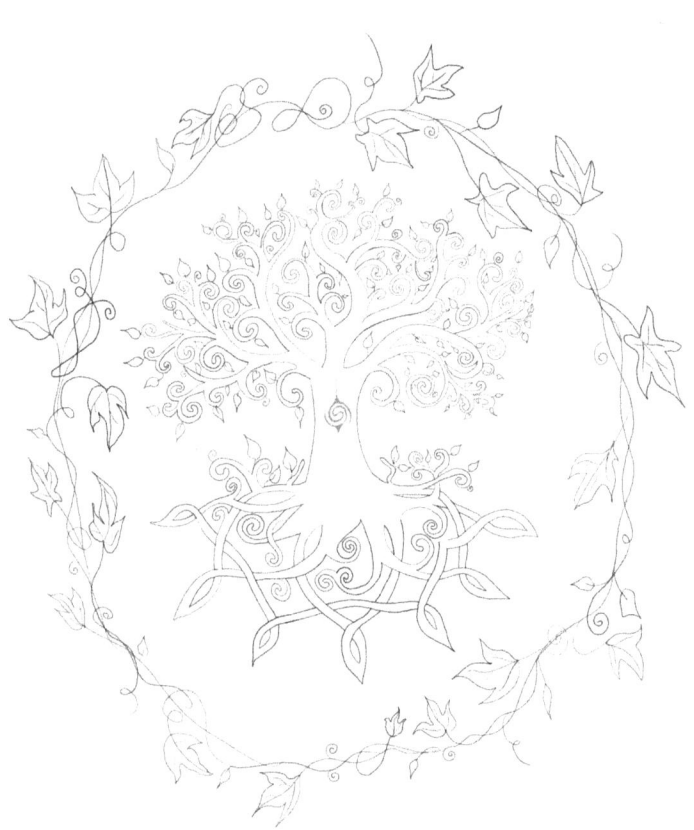

Recommended reading

Seasonal spirituality:

Cross, Emma-Jane: *Walking the Wheel of the Year.* Green Magic Publishing, UK, 2020.

Blake, Deborah; Connor, Kerri; Marquis, Melanie; Neal, Carl F.; Pesznecker, Susan; and Rajchel, Diana: *Llewellyn's Sabbat Essentials Series.* Llewellyn Worldwide, St. Paul, 2001.

Forest, Danu: *The Magical Year – Seasonal Celebrations to Honour Nature's Ever-Turning Wheel.* London: Watkins Publishing, London, 2016.

Hoff, Benjamin: *The Tao of Pooh.* Penguin Books, New York, 1983.

Kindred, Glennie: *The Earth's Cycle of Celebration.* G. Kindred, UK, 1994.

Kindred, Glennie; and Garner, Lu: *Creating Ceremony.* G. Kindred, UK, 1994.

Kindred, Glennie: *Elements of Change.* G. Kindred, UK, 1994.

Kindred, Glennie: *Earth Wisdom.* Hay House, London, 2005.

Murphy-Hiscock, Arin: *The House Witch.* Adams Media, 2018.

McCoy, Edain: *The Sabbats – A New Approach to Living the Old Ways.* Llewellyn Publications, St. Paul, 1999.

Moorey, T.; and Brideson, J.: *Wheel of the Year – Myth and Magic through the Seasons.* Hodder and Stoughton Educational, London, 1997.

Paxson, Diana L.: *Essential Asatru – Walking the Path of Norse Paganism.* Citadel, New York, 2006.

Redfield, James: *The Celestine Prophecy.* Bantam Books (Transworld Publishers, a division of the Random House Group), London, 1994.

Cookery Witch: https://www.youtube.com/@thewitchescookery

Historical:

Herbet, Kathleen: The Lost Gods of England. Anglo-Saxon Books, Ely, 1994.

Kondratiev, Alexi: *Celtic Rituals – An Authentic Guide to Ancient Celtic Spirituality*. Collins Press, Scotland, 1998.

Lindow, John: *Norse Mythology – A Guide to Gods, Heroes, Rituals and Beliefs*. Oxford University Press, 2001.

Pollington, Stephen: *The Elder Gods – The Otherworld of Early England*. Anglo-Saxon Books, Ely, 2011.

Stewart, R.J.: *Celtic Gods Celtic Goddesses*. Cassell Illustrated, London, 1990.

Wallis, Faith (trans.): *Bede – The Reckoning of Time*. Liverpool University Press, 1999.

Bibliography

Cross, Emma-Jane: *Walking the Wheel of the Year*. Green Magic Publishing, UK, 2020.

BrainFutures 2025 – Neuroplasticity 101: www.brainfutures.org/neuroplasticity-101

Ephemeris.com: History of Astronomy – The Celts, 2024: http://ephemeris.com/history/celts.html

Holmes, H.: A Rite of Passage – Tattie Holidays, 2016: https://blog.scottishagriculturalimplementmakers.co.uk/a-rite-of-passage-tattle-holidays/

Koosis, L.A.: The Science of Affirmations – The Brain's Response to Positive Thinking, 2024: https://www.mentalhealth.com/tools/science-of-affirmations

McShane, J.: What you should – and shouldn't – leave out for wildlife over winter, 2025: https://www.countryliving.com/uk/wildlife/countryside/a63480948/should-shouldnt-leave-out-wildlife-winter/

Siegel, R.D.: *The Mindfulness Solution – Everyday Practices for Everyday Problems*. The Guilford Press, New York, 2010.

Schwartz, D., PhD: *The Magic of Thinking Big*. New York: Touchstone Books, New York, 1987.

www.ingramcontent.com/pod-product-compliance
Lightning Source LLC
Chambersburg PA
CBHW061301110426
42742CB00012BA/2015